THE HEART OF HEALTH

The Principles of
Physical Health
and Vitality

by Stephen Linsteadt, N.D., C.N.C.
and Maria Elena Boekemeyer, N.D.

NATURAL
HEALING
HOUSE
PRESS

LIBRARY OF CONGRESS CATALOGING-IN-PUBLICATION DATA

Linstead, Stephen and Boekemeyer, Maria Elena.

The heart of health : principles of physical health and vitality /
by Stephen Linsteadt and Maria Elena Boekemeyer. —
1 st ed.
p. cm.
Includes bibliographical references.

ISBN 0-9741123-0-5

Library of Congress Control Number: 2003113203

The information contained in this book is intended for research and edu-
cational purposes only. The authors do not present any part of this work,
directly or indirectly, for the diagnoses or prescription of any disease or
condition. People who use the information from this book are advised to
take responsibility for consulting the health professional of their choice
regarding all matters pertaining to their physical, emotional or mental
health

Cover and Interior Design by Marilyn Hager Adleman
Editorial by Elizabeth Castaneda

Published by Natural Healing House Press
Grass Valley, California
http://www.naturalhealinghouse.com

Printed in the United States of America
by Central Plains Book Manufacturing

1 3 5 7 9 8 6 4 2

Contents

Foreword

This book is a must-read for anyone who wants an explanation of the extraordinary processes that support our well-being. Working with the basic principles that underlie health, Stephen Linsteadt and Maria Elena Boekemeyer detail the basic principles necessary for physical health and vitality and explain what prevents us from realizing this possibility.

I had the good fortune to experience the principles of health and vitality first hand when, after a life-time of vigorous health, I produced a miniscule .2 melanoma on my leg. I immediately went to see Stephen and Maria Elena and they quickly outlined the underlying cause. I had a massive infection in my jaw bone from toxic pus originating from 7 root canal teeth. The infection had depleted my immune and liver function. Because I had lived by stringent health practices for 30+ years, my immune system had managed to maintain its functioning in spite of my many root canal teeth. However, in the two years previous to my melanoma wake-up call I had broken some of the principles outlined in this book. I was over-worked, stressed and not getting sufficient sleep. With my defenses down, the root canal cysts and their toxic gases caught up with me. Stephen and Maria Elena provided me with dietary recommendations, an individualized supplement and detoxification program and German biological remedies. The medical doctor they work with prescribed a substance that I used on my leg that selectively kills tumor cells without harming healthy cells. Three weeks after my visit with Stephen and Maria Elena I returned to see them and to have the remaining surrounding tissue removed from my leg. This was a precautionary measure because the doctor who did the original biopsy was certain she had left melanoma cells at the site of the procedure and insisted that follow-up surgery was essential for everyone's peace of mind. A biopsy of the follow-up procedure showed no signs of melanoma.

The other happy result of going to see Stephen and Maria Elena was that we discussed the principles of physical vitality and health and our mutual desire to write a book about the whole spectrum of what makes physical vitality and a high state of health possible. We also wanted to provide a practical program, which would organize how to put the principles into action, especially for people with busy lives.

I am thrilled that Stephen and Maria Elena have agreed to synthesize their knowledge and experience in this book for the benefit of our health. I am also excited to share my own experience and program in my book, *Brush with Death, Commitment to Life: a Program for Super- Health and Vitality*. This program is the "Principles" in action and is the companion to this book. Our hope is that these two books together will help people understand the principles and daily practice of optimal physical health and thereby experience the joy of living unlimited potential.

Chloe Faith Wordsworth

Author of, *Brush with Death, Commitment to Life:*
A Program for Super Health and Vitality

Introduction

This book explains many of the reasons why we become sick while providing meaningful advice on how to stay young and healthy. The concepts delineated here are what we refer to as the Principles of Physical Health and Vitality.

This book is for those that want to understand the basic natural laws of staying healthy. It is a guide, a road map, to show you how you can take control of your own health in order to reach the natural balance that leads to optimal physical health and vitality. This book lays out the basics of energy and nutritional medicine. It shows how these two powerful healing tools/concepts intertwine to become the "Heart of Health."

Vitality is perhaps new to many people. Vitality is not a physical attribute. It is a feeling of well-being and the energy that comes from having optimal physical health. It is also the sense of high mental and emotional coherence. Coherence is the opposite of chaos. When our thoughts are chaotic and negative our cells also become less coherent and de-energized. Our thoughts and emotions play a big role in the status of our physical health. Often it is our desire to control outside events that moves us away from our inner peace and gives rise to negative thoughts and feelings. Therefore, to achieve optimal physical health, we have to start with our mental and emotional well-being, the basis of which is faith in ourselves. Having an inner connection and love for ourselves can help us overcome health challenges and feelings of hopelessness during the most difficult periods of our lives.

Having faith in a higher source or at least in the power of our higher self, opens the door to achieving higher possibilities. When we surrender our sense of 'self' and instead see ourselves as a part of the Divine plan, we see only the positive in everything that happens. This allows us to stop focussing on the negative or on those things that we cannot change or control. Instead, we see setbacks in our lives as positive opportunities for deep personal growth. When we possess firm faith in ourselves, we find the mental and emotional well-being that generates the positive energy that leads us to optimal physical health. We have VITALITY. We are FULLY alive, radiant, and joyful. We simply feel good about ourselves and we WANT to take care of ourselves. We naturally want to do things that are life enhancing. We find that we select nutritious wholesome foods. We feel like exercising. And, our relationships with our spouse, children and those around us are more harmonious. Everything that we do is life-enhancing and coherent.

Inner and Outer Connection

When we are truly in tune to ourselves we are also connected to everyone around us. The question is: What is it that we are all connected to? Scientists have shown that at the fundamental sub-atomic level of our being, we are only energy. The source of this energy is unknown, but it is there just the same.

Scientists have demonstrated that all cells receive, store and emit quantum packets of light, called bio-photons.[1] These biophotons are stored and released from within the helical structure of the DNA molecule, which when unwound measures seven feet long.[2,3] This DNA molecule acts like an antenna to receive light energy from the solar system, from the universe, from the cosmic energy that gives us life.

This subtle unifying energy (the quantum field) is the most fundamental level of energy. It cascades into outer layers of increasing densities of energy until it eventually reaches the electromagnetic domain that we see captured and stored within our DNA. These electromagnetic fields regulate and control all biochemical and biological processes.[4]

Contemporary cell research is now based on the principles of quantum physics that shows the world as being created out of energy. Researchers have now demonstrated that our cells' membranes contain special proteins called Intergral Membrane Proteins (IMPs) that respond to energy signals from the external and internal environment. These are important findings because they acknowledge that biological behavior can be controlled by "invisible" energy forces, which include thought.[5]

When we shut off our internal mind-talk and concentrate our attention through prayer, meditation or contemplation, we tune ourselves into this subtle, spiritual, quantum-level energy matrix. When this energy is allowed to transfer to our DNA (without interruption from negative attitudes), it affects the molecular and cellular levels that drive all our physical metabolic processes. This is why we have the ability to heal ourselves through prayer, meditation or conscious intention.

We are all connected to each other and to the energy source that makes up the universe. We are totally inter-dependent. Our body, our brain, our consciousness are inextricably joined with other matter in the universe. Every atom and molecule within us depends on the rest of the universe. Our brain and other parts of our neural physiology are interconnected by this unseen communication network which coordinates and regulates behavior of certain parts of the body.[6] The body, therefore, can be seen as a dense medium holding the real essence of who we are—Divine energy. We are interconnected outward expressions of this Divine energy. This interconnection is all-pervasive and instantaneous. The manifestation of this energy comes from the 'empty' vacuum, known as the quantum vacuum, which is actually 'packed full' of God's creative energy in a stable state. This all-pervading energy is sometimes referred to as a universal scalar wave, which is a form of electrostatic energy that has the potential to create but is currently without physical manifestation. Potential is only manifested when we provide the frequency information through our thoughts and intentions of what it is we want to create. This is the concept of 'mind over matter.' Our potential is unlimited and therefore what we are capable of creating is also unlimited.

The energetic link that we all share explains how our intentions, thoughts and prayers can travel to a sick friend and connect with their mind and consciousness. It also explains why every action is followed by a reaction. Everything that happens to one particle or to a collection of particles, as in our being, affects every other particle. All of our actions and thoughts have ramifications throughout the universe.

A collection of cells is what makes up 'ourselves,' in the same way as a collection of 'ourselves' makes up a society. Therefore, our relationship with others is, in fact, having a relationship with ourselves. We are the same. We are from the same source. This is why the people in our lives are always pushing our buttons. They are a mirror to us of who 'we' are. When we don't like what we see, it is 'us' that we are having a problem with.

The body is also constantly generating these universal scalar waves. Scalar waves are produced when two electromagnetic waves of the same frequency are exactly out of phase (opposite to each other) and the amplitudes subtract and cancel or destroy each other. The result is not exactly an annihilation of magnetic fields but a transformation of energy back into a scalar wave. This scalar field has reverted back to a vacuum state of potentiality. Scalar waves can be created by wrapping electrical wires around a figure eight in the shape of a möbius coil. When an electric current flows through the wires in opposite directions, the opposing electromagnetic fields from the two wires cancel each other and create a scalar wave.

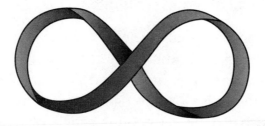

The DNA antenna in our cells' energy production centers (mitochondria) assumes the shape of what is called a super-coil.[3] Supercoil DNA look like a series of möbius coils. These möbius supercoil DNA are hypothetically able to generate scalar waves. Most cells in the body contain thousands of these möbius supercoils, which are generating scalar waves throughout the cell and throughout the body.

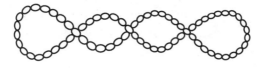

There is another möbius coil configuration found within the vascular system. The continuous flow of blood through the arterial system—which runs next to the venous system but in opposite directions—contains möbius coil properties. The circulation of blood throughout the body resembles the figure-eight shape of the möbius coil. Within the vascular möbius coil there are subsets of the figure eight along the major capillary networks. These major capillary networks are associated with primary organs and are related to the endocrine glands.

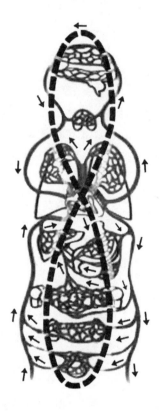

The electrical activity of the heart muscle sets up its electromagnetic field, the strongest field of the body. It is at the heart that the center of the vascular möbius coil is found: an intersection of venous blood passing through the right atrium, overlapping aortic blood coming through the left atrium. The möbius coil intersection occurs just in front of

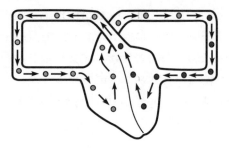

the lungs, which contain a huge web-like network of capillary connections. This capillary network acts as a battery for the storage of scalar waves.

Scalar waves generated in the body protect us from the negative effects of solar radiation and other environmental electromagnetic stresses by constantly producing a neutral field capable of deflecting these harmful non-bioenergetically compatible frequencies. Scalar waves generated in the body also provide an energetic communication system that connects all cells. This energy contains the power of the universe and has unlimited potential.

In the scalar vacuum state this energy is susceptible to our thoughts and feelings. Our cells react to environmental signals as well as to our thoughts. Cells move toward growth signals and away from life-threatening stimuli.[7] Cells naturally move outwardly in growth and replication but are forced to retract or conserve their energy when repairing or feeling attacked. A cell cannot be in growth and protection mode at the same time. If our tissues and organs perceive a need for protection due to our negative thoughts, they will compromise their growth behavior.[7] Chronic protection leads to a disruption of the tissue and its function.[7] Our positive mental attitude is communicated through the scalar field generated by thousands of möbius coils at the cellular level and can effect the cell's mode of growth or protection. Scientists have created scalar wave generators for therapeutic purposes and have confirmed that a scalar field can create a twenty-fold stimulation of cell growth in human immune system cells.[4]

The ability of the body to produce scalar waves may not be new news. Notice the similarity between the DNA supercoil and the Caduceus Staff below. Is it possible that "Healers" from antiquity knew about the remarkable healing property of the möbius coil?

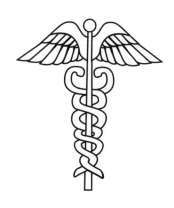

Positive Mental and Emotional Attitude

Thoughts and emotions have an electromagnetic frequency vibration that is perceived by every cell in the body through the instant communication system of scalar waves. Negative thoughts and emotions can interfere with the electromagnetic, biophoton signaling at the cellular membrane and DNA levels. When this happens, the communication signals become chaotic and cellular information and instructions for enzyme and protein formation become blocked. The same thing happens when you are trying to get a clear picture on your television set. The TV antenna must be pointed in the direction of the transmitted incoming signal. Without this focussing you only get static. When you turn your attention away from the source (the Spirit or quantum energy source) by focusing on negative thoughts and emotions, your cells and DNA receive and transmit static. In this case, your cells lose the signal or instructions on what to do and they become chaotic or uneasy, as in 'dis-ease.'

If you look at the source of negative thoughts and emotions, in all cases you will find that the root cause is "fear." When you allow fear to interfere (enter-fear) with your DNA signaling, you are traveling down the path of cellular degeneration. The opposite of fear is love. Unconditional love is the emotional quality or feeling associated with having a connection with the "Universal Creative Energy." Love is the highest positive energy. It transcends all other feelings and emotions. Love is the energy and power of God or the Source of what keeps us alive. When we are connected to the highest expression of love, there is no room for fear. With love there is trust—trust in our abilities and ourselves; trust in the Divine plan. You can love someone without trusting them, but you cannot have trust without love. Having fear means you have become out of step with Trust and Love.

To remedy this, the first step is to identify the negative thought or emotion. What is it you are thinking about that weakens you and disrupts your DNA communication system? What is the situation or person that causes this reaction in you? The way we react to an event is recorded in our molecular matrix. If each cell contains all of the information for the whole organism, then our experiences, good or bad, are also recorded on a cellular level. Those experiences that we perceive as life threatening may continue to resonate within the memory banks of the body's crystalline cellular and molecular matrix because we were not able to resolve the conflict or dissipate its energy. This matrix memory can alter our beliefs about ourselves and consequently our behavior as a result of the earlier, traumatic experience. This can cause us to feel disempowered, have low self-esteem, or feel unloved. These feelings all have a resonant frequency signature that vibrates throughout our being. This energetic disturbance can upset neurohormonal pathways in our body and constrict the energetic flow to cells, DNA, organ tissue, muscle tissue, and other systems in our body. When we can identify the source of the upset and reduce it to the underlying fear, we take the first step towards shifting the fear into trust. This can be as simple as changing the channel on your television set. If you don't like what you are watching you can always grab the remote and change the channel to something more uplifting. Likewise, we can change the channel of what we think about and the external conditions also change. Once we change then our spouse, child, friend, or the negative situation can change next. Just change the channel of what you and your DNA resonate with and you change your reality. It is like two prisoners gazing out from behind bars —one sees mud and the other sees stars. We have the choice about what we believe about ourselves. Our positive self-image defines what we become.

Often we are not able to identify the upset or past trauma. In this case, it may not be as easy as just changing the channel of our thoughts. Even though many of these issues have been long forgotten, subconsciously, our behavior is still shaped by them. Our molecular and cellular matrix remembers the painful experience and may cause us to avoid situations that seem similar for fear of reenacting the experience. Poor health often results. In addition, this constricted energy many times affects our habits and perceptions in negative ways. For example, often our misperceptions lead us to actions that create obstacles that keep us from achieving our highest possibilities. We develop unworkable relationships due to negative actions or we block our professional goals because of low self-esteem. Our beliefs about ourselves sabotage our creativity and general well-being.

Chloe Faith Wordsworth developed a system called "Holographic Repatterning," that safely identifies these emotional trauma patterns in our energy matrix. This process uses a 'strong' muscle indicator response or a 'weak' muscle indicator response to systematically identify the unresolved subconscious conflicts that cause negative behavior. A series of strong and weak muscle indicator responses provides a holographic picture of the inner conflicts that influence our behavior in sometimes self-sabotaging ways.

Once identified, these negative emotional patterns can be released from the system by using various energetic techniques aimed at the specific energy frequency that needs to be dissipated or repatterned. Once you let go of the emotional distress, your thoughts and actions are no longer influenced by subconscious self-sabotaging influences. The unresolved earlier traumatic experience finds resolution and the negative mind talk is replaced with a positive outlook. This allows for a new internal motivation where life becomes meaningful and you have a clear sense of purpose. Without the influence of the negative patterns from the past you harmoniously resolve differences in your relationships. Problems are seen as opportunities for growth and improvement. You're empowered by challenges. You respond to life with trust, confidence, calmness, courage and positive action. You feel energized and have a sense of physical well-being.[8]

One common modality or energetic tool used in Holographic Repatterning is Quantum Healing Codes. The codes are a series of five frequencies or notes discovered by Dr. Puleo as outlined in his book, *Healing Codes—for the Biological Apocalypse*. They are based on the idea that there exists a predictable geometric pattern behind all matter. All matter owes its existence to vibrating frequencies. The vibrating energy of various frequencies is behind the energetic blueprint that governs all of the molecular and biochemical processes of our bodies.

The events of our past can leave an energetic imprint on our emotional, mental and physical bodies in such a way as to become the subconscious motivator of our current day behavior. These discordant frequencies can also become lodged in the crystalline structure of our tissue and reverberate within the water molecules that make up over 65 percent of our body. These discordant frequencies can create areas of non-coherence that lead to obstructions between the body's energetic and cellular communication systems. The breakdown of healthy frequency information can lead to weakened immunity, less than optimal organ, nervous system, brain, hormonal, and skeletal functions as well as chronic pain.

The phenomenon of resonance can be dramatically experienced by the example of the opera singer who hits a high enough note as to exactly match the same resonant frequency of a nearby glass. This results in the molecules holding the glass together vibrating so strongly that the glass shatters. This same phenomenon can occur within our bodies. When we say that we don't resonate with someone, we are really saying that the vibratory energy of that person vibrates an uncomfortable chord within ourselves. They may be striking a chord that resonates with a traumatic experience we had with someone as a child. The vibratory energy of these early experiences that are lodged within our tissue can be excited and activated even by the smallest subconscious reminder.

In Holographic Repatterning the earlier experience is identified along with the area of the body/mind system that is holding on to the frequency information of the event. In order to release this vibratory frequency once and for all there are many energetic techniques used to cancel out these discordant frequencies. The use of audible sound frequencies is one such modality. Some have used tuning forks with much success in this area. The use of two tuning forks can be even more powerful due to the fact that you can create dissonant chords or intervals by using two or more 'notes'. The use of dissonant chords can resonate with the painful early experience and shatter it from our molecular memory.

Quantum Healing Codes are used to reestablish coherence within our body/mind system by shattering limiting and painful experiences as well as bringing greater coherence to the system with powerful healing frequencies. The codes are used to diffuse those patterns that are life depleting and to create patterns that are life enhancing. This tool helps transform non-coherent energy patterns that arise from a cellular memory of a past trauma.

If you identify with having negative thoughts or emotions you may refer to the last chapter entitled Scalar Heart Connection. This simple exercise may help you transform these negative frequencies into positive, life-enhancing vibrations. If you find that you need to go even deeper into the source of your limiting patterns, you may need to have someone more objective than yourself help you identify and shift these old negative beliefs. Holographic Repatterning is one such tool. More information on Holographic Repatterning is available in the resource section at the end of this book.

Physical Ecology (pH)

The physical body represents the densest configuration of energy. How this energy manifests on the physical cellular level is determined by the subtle energy that flows from our thoughts and feelings. Our thoughts and negative attitudes interfere with how our cells communicate with each other and how we communicate with others. It is the frequency vibrations arising from our subtle energy blueprint that holds all of the atoms and molecules of our body together.

Our body is made up of only cells. The body contains a hundred trillion cells. There are 300 million new cells built every minute.[9] All of our cells are made up of atoms. The synthesis of each protein that makes up the structure of our body requires a half dozen or more steps—totaling hundreds of thousands, even billions, of reactions occurring every moment. All of these cellular processes involve a flow and transport of electrons or protons. It is this flow of atomic particles that provides the micro-electric currents that are responsible for all of our biochemical processes. The frequency vibrations from our subtle energy matrix travel through the body along cell membranes, through bi-polar water molecule chains, along protein chains, and through the electrolyte-rich connective tissue, reaching every nook and corner of the body.

The quality of these communication pathways is critical in determining the quality of information transfer and the flow of micro-electric currents throughout the body. This ultra-fine bio-electric energy is found in our nervous system, brain activity, muscles, heart function, etc. and is dependent on an adequate supply of minerals to conduct electricity. These minerals, calcium, sodium, potassium, phosphate, chloride and magnesium are called electrolytes. The body requires different electrolyte concentrations in blood plasma, tissues, and cellular fluid for the flow of bio-electricity.

Bio-electricity must be able to pass freely throughout the body in order for cellular processes and communications to function properly. When we do not have the proper amount of electrolytes in our body cellular signaling is interrupted. Inter-cellular communication occurs throughout the extracellular tissue matrix. This matrix contains electrolytes and other substances. These fluids are our physical ecology, our cellular environment.

Within our internal ecology our bloodstream and lymphatic system act like a stream that is an environment or ecosystem for frogs, fish and plant life. In order to avoid an ecological disaster, the acid/alkaline (pH) balance of the stream has to be just right or the water gets murky and full of germs. In such a polluted lake frogs may be born with five legs and three eyes, while plant life withers and the adjacent soil erodes. The whole eco-system dies. In the same way, our watery internal environment has to have a proper pH balance. If our internal ecology becomes polluted or stagnant, the entire eco-system, microorganisms as well as the body's tissues and organs are also affected. In such a polluted body microorganisms that ordinarily live synergistically (helpfully and harmoniously) inside our body mutate and become pathogenic or disease producing.

Our internal ecology requires a slightly alkaline pH ("Potential of Hydrogen") in order to provide adequate oxygen levels for optimal cellular functioning and a clean internal environment. PH is a measure of the relative acidity or alkalinity of a solution. A pH of 7.0 is neutral (pure water is 7.0).

pH Scale of Acidic Reactions

ACID		ALKALINE	
0 1 2 3 4 5 6	7	8 9 10 11 12 13 14	

An optimal pH for the blood is slightly alkaline at 7.35 to 7.45 due to the presence of electrolytes. Electrolytes are alkaline elements. These alkaline minerals are responsible for the transmission of bio-electricity in our body and for nerve communication. They also act to neutralize the acids that are produced from the food we eat as well as from the acid by-products or the waste the body produces.

Normal pH Ranges

Gastric	1.00 – 3.50
Duodenum	4.20 – 8.20
Urine	4.80 – 5.80
Saliva	6.50 – 7.50
Liver Bile	7.10 – 8.50
Pancreas	8.00 – 8.30
Blood	7.35 – 7.45

The chart below shows that there is a big difference between the acidity of the gastric acids in the stomach (from 1.00 to 3.50) to the acidity found in the intestines (from 4.20 all the way up to an alkaline pH of 8.20). The pancreas, which secretes many of the enzymes needed for digestion and assimilation, can only work at a pH of 8.00 to 8.30.

Functioning pH Ranges

	1.0	1.5	2.0	2.5	3.0	3.5	4.0	4.5	5.0	5.5	6.0	6.5	7.0	7.5	8.0
Gastric	█	█	█	█	█	█									
Duodenum							█	█	█	█	█	█	█	█	
Urine							█	█	█						
Saliva												█	█	█	
Liver Bile													█	█	█
Pancreas															█
Blood													█	█	

The stomach acid, hydrochloric acid, is derived from the element chlorine (hydrogen and chloride: hydrochloric-acid). Hydrochloric acid in the stomach is our first line of defense against invading bacteria and parasites. Hydrochloric acid also aids in the digestion of protein. When we eat more acid forming foods (meat, bread) than alkaline forming foods (vegetables) we deplete our store of alkalizing electrolyte minerals such as sodium bicarbonate. One of the results of a loss of alkaline-buffering reserves is that the body slows down the production of hydrochloric acid. This not only compromises our ability to digest food, protein in particular, but also impairs our ability to defend ourselves against pathogens.

Under normal conditions, the acidic content of the stomach is released into the first part of the small intestines, known as the duodenum. The gallbladder releases bile, which is produced by the liver, and mixes with alkaline pancreatic juices in order to reduce the acidic stomach contents to an alkaline level suitable for the digestive enzymes to finish the job of digestion and assimilation.

When we constantly eat acidic-forming foods, over time we deplete our alkaline reserves and the enzymes from the pancreas can't fully break the food down. Partially digested food particles continue to travel down the 25 feet of intestines where they putrefy and rot. Putrefying food upsets the delicate intestinal flora (good microorganisms) and often activates an overgrowth of candida, which results in constipation, bloating, headaches, and gas.

When the gallbladder and pancreas are not able to supply sufficient alkaline buffering minerals to the duodenum the pH sensitive intestines can't accept the acidic stomach contents. The pyloric sphincter, which separates the stomach from the first part of the small intestines (duodenum), is pH sensitive—meaning that it does not release the acidic stomach contents unless it also senses the correct alkaline pH on the other side. This is Nature's way of ensuring that we don't damage the delicate intestinal tissue. Unfortunately, the unpleasant side effect of the pyloric valve not accepting the stomach contents is that the contents can back up into the stomach and cause heartburn. If the problem is severe enough the stomach contents can be sent right out from where they came.

The depletion of alkaline reserves in the gallbladder and pancreas causes the body to attempt to pull alkaline electrolyte minerals from calcium in the bloodstream and bones. However, as the chart above illustrates, our blood must be slightly alkaline at 7.35 to 7.45. If our blood is higher or lower than this range the bio-electricity to the heart will be interrupted and we will die. Therefore, the body will do everything possible to maintain this narrow alkaline range of the blood. It will even take the alkaline sodium, potassium and chloride salts from the gallbladder reserves to neutralize an overly acidic bloodstream. When the gallbladder is depleted in alkaline reserves and is also looking for additional support there is no choice except to draw upon the calcium in the bones to supply the bloodstream as well as the digestive system.

When the gallbladder is forced to give up its alkaline salt contents to the blood to maintain the correct pH of the blood, cholesterol naturally found in liquid form in the gallbladder becomes solid. This leads to the formation of gallstones. When the gallbladder becomes congested with gallstones the flow of bile from the liver is restricted. When this happens the toxins from the liver cannot be eliminated through the intestines and are instead passed on to the kidneys. When the kidneys can no longer handle the flow of poisonous toxins the excess is passed to the skin for elimination or stored within the joints and connective tissue. A liver congested due to gallstones can cause nausea, diarrhea, constipation, hernias, hemorrhoids, breathing difficulties, hepatitis, high cholesterol, pancreatitis, heart disease, brain disorders, duodenal ulcers, urinary problems, prostate diseases, hormonal imbalances, loss of vision, headaches, skin disorders, liver spots, osteoporosis, chronic fatigue, kidney diseases, and cancer.

Instead of detoxifying the gallbladder by natural means and balancing the pH through diet, most people automatically have their gallbladder surgically removed. In some circumstances this may be a life-saving procedure as a ruptured gallbladder leads to death. However, nature provides plenty of warning signs that the gallbladder is in need of a thorough cleans.

When the alkaline balance is upset, the intestinal fungi take over, the colon absorbs their toxic by-products and sends them directly to the liver. The liver enzymes needed to break-down these toxins are also sensitive to a narrow pH range and cannot function optimally without an alkaline pH. As a result, toxins from the liver are not fully broken down for elimination through the intestines but instead, the liver passes them off into the bloodstream, where they cause the blood to become too acidic.

If our blood and tissues are constantly in a dangerously acidic condition, the gallbladder runs low on alkaline minerals and the pancreatic enzymes become deactivated. In this case, our entire digestive process becomes compromised and we begin to suffer from malabsorption of essential vitamins, minerals and other nutrients. Without adequate nutrients and important vitamins, other metabolic processes become impaired and toxins begin to build up. This leads to physical problems as well as depression, anxiety, worry, grief and general feelings of unhappiness that cause us to fall out of sync with our inner and outer connection. Our communication systems break down.

Now we have a degenerative loop. The acidic blood tries to compensate by taking alkaline salts from the gallbladder, which has been surgically removed, or is under-functioning because of its own toxic buildup. This forces the blood to borrow alkaline minerals (i.e., calcium) from the bones, jaw and teeth. The consequences are bleeding gums, weak and broken hips, knee problems and osteoporosis.

Over time, the entire body, including cellular and extra cellular fluids, becomes acidic. Acidity repels oxygen. A lack of oxygen lowers the energy production in our oxygen dependent cells. The microbes in our blood also depend on oxygen for their energy production and sustenance. A lack of oxygen causes them to change their metabolism to an anaerobic, non-oxygen dependent metabolism. The by-products of an anaerobic metabolism are toxic to healthy cells. This creates a situation where the once friendly microorganisms are now pathogenic and potentially harmful. This in turn strains our immune system.

A combination of low oxygen, poor and toxic circulation, and a weak immune system are the pre-requisites for cancer and other chronic illnesses.

Negative thoughts stimulate acidic conditions in the stomach or duodenum. Anger, bitterness, hate, jealousy, grudges, and other negative feelings, attitudes and expressions produce vibrations that influence the body chemistry and glandular functions. When we loose our inner balance and connection we tend to be chronically anxious or plagued with inner emotional turmoil or habitually find events around us upsetting. This keeps the body on "survival mode," which leads to increased levels of adrenal hormones in response to stress. The adrenal stress hormones are acid producing and suppress the digestive system which affects the amount of enzymes that are produced, the quantity of bile available and intestinal activity. The adrenal stress response also plays a role in the suppression of hydrochloric acid production in the stomach. For these reasons, our emotional state and our inner and outer connection have a direct effect on the kind of bacteria that grow in the intestines and the amount of intestinal toxicity present. In turn, the amount of bacteria and toxicity levels affect our emotional well-being. This becomes a degenerative loop.

One way to find out if you are acidic and potentially on the path to a degenerative illness, is to do a very simple test. Leave a piece of litmus paper (pH paper available at your local pharmacy) on your bed stand at night and test your saliva pH before you get out of bed in the morning. This will tell you the pH status of your extracellular fluid. The pH reading should be 6.8 or higher (more alkaline). If the pH reading is less (more acidic), then you are compromising all of the chemical processes that take place in your body.

Measuring the pH of the urine is another method but can be misleading. Normally, we want to have urine that is slightly acidic because the urine is the route of elimination for toxic and acidic waste products. Some people become overjoyed when they test their urine and get a reading of 7.5 or 8.0. What they don't realize is that their system is so acidic that the body has lost all alkaline reserves and has to take the emergency measure of utilizing ammonia, which is very alkaline, in order to protect the urinary track from being damaged by the otherwise acidic urine. Urine that is alkaline as a result of ammonia indicates that you are in serious trouble.[10]

Hormone Balance

Hormones are another communication system in the body. Hormones are chemicals secreted by various endocrine glands that travel through the bloodstream to remote areas of the body where they have powerful controlling effects. They act like little messengers that carry signals throughout the body communicating instructions that synchronize cellular function, regeneration and repair of the entire body.

Hormones are molecules mostly produced by enzymes and bio-active proteins along with vitamins and minerals derived from our food. A smaller group of hormones known as steroids are produced by the adrenal and the sex organs and are formed largely from cholesterol and essential fatty acids. The pH range for optimal hormone production and activity is between 6.8 and 7.4.[11]

Hormones have specific shapes and dock to hormone receptor sites on the cell membrane in a lock and key configuration. There are also hormone receptor sites within the cell. Hormones create a chemical interaction at the cell membrane that stimulates the cell to perform specific functions or to turn off specific activities. These molecules also contain specific energetic vibrations. Through their specific frequency oscillations hormones are able to send

vibrations of information and instructions to distant tar-
geted cells and organs. Resonant receptors receive this
information like a radio receiving the news. Hormones,
therefore, can be seen as the interface between the electromagnetic and the bio-chemical energy states. The subtle
and unifying Universal energy acts like a blueprint that
guides and directs molecules. The body's bio-electrical
energy, which is derived from these molecular configura-
tions, gives rise to all bio-chemical reactions and processes
that we see in the hormonal communication and control
system.

Physical health and vitality depend on an efficient communication and regulation system. The hormonal system
depends on having an adequate number of messengers.
One of the most important hormone messengers is Human
Growth Hormone (HGH). HGH is produced by the pituitary gland and is responsible for sending signals to our
cells to grow. It is involved with all regulation, regeneration and cell replacement. Adequate levels of HGH help to
decrease fat and increase muscle mass even into old age.
Another particularly important hormone is DHEA (dehy-
droepiniandrosterone). It is an anti-stress hormone and is
the precursor to all sex hormones. HGH and DHEA give
us vitality and help us to stay and feel young.

A third important hormone is melatonin. It is produced primarily by the pineal gland. It is capable of permeating any
cell in any part of the body and protects the nucleus of the
cell against damage to its DNA. Low melatonin levels have
been correlated with multiple sclerosis, coronary artery disease, epilepsy, and post-menopausal osteoporosis.[12]

As we age the production of hormones can decline by 10 percent per decade. However, it is not always the case that we lose the ability to produce hormones as we age. Rather, we often lack the nutrients and enzymes needed to convert basic hormones into active hormones or we do not maintain an alkaline pH. In either case, the enzymes necessary for hormone production become deactivated.

As we saw earlier, when we are acidic we are not able to fully digest our food, and therefore we do not fully absorb the nutrients we need for hormone production. For example, the essential fatty acids from omega 3 and 6 oils help to produce eicosanoid hormones. These fats contain linoleic acid (LA), which is enzymatically converted to gamma linoleic acid (GLA). GLA is rarely found in food and therefore must be produced in the body. The enzyme required for the conversion of LA to GLA is only activated under an alkaline pH.

These fatty acids are important because they form powerful hormones. These hormones in turn affect the energy flow throughout the body, cell division, and immune system responses. They also make up the cell membrane, and determine the integrity of our nerve cells.

Some signs of omega 6 deficiency are high blood pressure, PMS or breast pain, eczema or dry skin, inflammatory problems (arthritis), diabetes, multiple sclerosis, mental health problems, or excessive thirst. Signs of omega 3 deficiency includes dry skin, inflammation, tingling in the arms or legs, high blood pressure, high triglycerides (fat in the blood), frequent infections, inability to lose weight, memory loss, learning disability, lack of coordination, or impaired vision.

The most important thing to remember is that the body receives "good" essential oils (omega 3 and 6) from the leaves of plants and their seeds. Sunflower seeds, pumpkin seeds, and flax seeds are good examples.

It is also important to remember that excessive intake of essential oils can accelerate aging unless you also increase your consumption of antioxidants, such as vitamin E, C, zinc, magnesium, and selenium. You will see why later.

In addition to maintaining an alkaline pH and obtaining proper essential fatty acids and pre-cursor nutrients, it is also important that we reduce the amount of toxins in our body. Circulating toxins from the environment or from poor food choices can damage hormone receptor sites or block communication pathways. Healthy hormone function depends on adequate levels of hormones in the system and working receptor sites at the target cells. And, the hormone communication system must be toxin free to allow hormones to pass through the bloodstream to find their targets. For this reason the health of the liver is vital because the liver is responsible for the purification of the bloodstream.

The liver does more than just breakdown toxins. The liver also plays a role in hormone production. As we saw earlier, one of the most important hormones for maintaining youthful health and vitality is Human Growth Hormone. However, HGH is not the hormone that actually performs all of these beneficial functions. The liver first absorbs

HGH, where it is converted into another hormone called IGF-1 (short for Insulin-like Growth Factor). IGF-1 is the active form of HGH that is actually responsible for the effects attributed to HGH. If the liver is full of toxins then this very important conversion activity is disrupted, and we miss out on the cellular growth promoting benefits of HGH/IGF-1. The consequence is cellular degeneration that we view as the normal process of aging or worse, the beginning of chronic illness.

In addition, if the liver is overburdened with toxins it is not able to produce cholesterol. Cholesterol, produced by the liver, is used by the cell's energy factories to create a hormone called pregnenolone. Pregnenolone is made primarily in the adrenal glands, but is also produced in the liver and brain. Pregnenolone is an important hormone because it is the building block for DHEA, progesterone, and the adrenal stress hormones. DHEA, as we saw earlier, is an important anti-stress hormone and a precursor to all of the sex hormones. The production of DHEA is particularly important for post-menopausal women as the adrenal gland production of DHEA helps to make up for the loss of estrogen and progesterone from the ovaries. Sufficient amounts of DHEA can elevate the symptoms of menopause and help maintain healthful levels of estrogen and progesterone.

Under normal conditions the liver is able to keep up with the onslaught of toxins introduced by the food we eat and from environmental pollution. The liver uses a group of enzymes, referred to as cytochrome P450 enzymes to metabolize these toxins. This enzyme system is important in neutralizing cellular toxins. These enzymes are responsible for neutralizing such toxins as caffeine, alcohol and other wastes that are absorbed by the intestines. These same enzymes also play a role in the conversion of pregnenolone into DHEA and the other hormones mentioned above.

The cytochrome P450 enzymes are also sensitive to pH and require an alkaline environment in order to function properly. Therefore, in order to maintain optimal levels of youth promoting hormones, we need to reduce our intake of acid promoting food and reduce our exposure to toxins.

The liver requires a constant supply of the precursor nutrients that go into the making of these cytochrome P450 enzymes, such as vitamin C, magnesium, copper, zinc, niacin, thiamin and iron. Therefore, it is essential that we eat a diet that supplies adequate levels of these nutrients. From the chart below we can see how important it is to maintain a healthy liver as it is involved in many important functions.

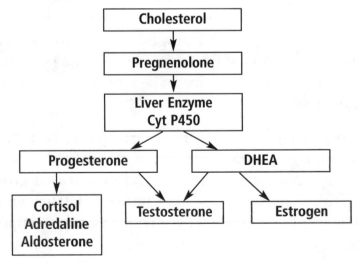

Hormone and pH - Enhancing Foods
(When eaten in a ratio of 80% alkaline and 20% acidic)

Vegetables (alkaline)
Spinach
Chard
Kale
Broccoli
Brussels Sprouts
Cauliflower
Cabbage Barley
Parsley
Green Peas
Zucchini
Green Beans
Cucumbers
Green Peppers
Artichokes
Celery
Tomatoes
Onions
Beets
Carrots
Corn

Fruit (alkaline)
Apples
Pears
Peaches
Grapes
Grapefruit
Bananas
Oranges
Lemons

Grains (acidic)
Wheat Germ (raw)
Wheat Berries (red)
Wild Rice
Whole Brown Rice
Oatmeal (steel cut)
Millet (alkaline)

Nuts and Seeds (raw)
Sesame Seeds (alkaline)
Almonds (pre-soaked) (alkaline)
Cashews (acidic)
Pumpkin (alkaline)

Legumes (acidic)
Lentils
Mung Beans (neutral)
Split Peas
Kidney Beans
Lima Beans (alkaline)
Garbanzo Beans

Oils – EFA's
Flaxseed (raw–cold pressed)
Evening Primrose (raw-CP)
Olive (cold pressed, extra Virgin)
Avocado

Cellular Nutrition

The trillions of cells that make up our body reflect our positive mental and emotional outlook and our connection with our inner sense of self-worth and self-confidence. This connection provides a coherent energetic blueprint for the body's communication network. When we are coherent and harmonious our cells are able to communicate via DNA signaling and hormone messengering. The cellular level is the most dense of energetic levels. It is the culmination of the subtle energy level, the molecular level, and the bio-energetic/bio-chemical level. It is at the physical cellular level that we live and express who we are. These trillions of cells require nutrients to carry out all of their billions of metabolic processes. In order to function at optimum levels, cells require specific micronutrients in exact proportions and ratios. These nutrients supply the cells with the ingredients they need to make proteins, to generate energy and to perform other physiological tasks like digestion, respiration, circulation, etc.

In addition to these essential tasks, cells also utilize various substances and nutrients to protect themselves against the harmful effects of oxygen known as oxidative stress. You may already be familiar with some everyday examples of this type of reaction: iron rusting, cut apples turning brown, and butter going rancid—these are all examples of the effects of oxidation reactions.

Oxidation reactions occur at the atomic level. Most stable molecules that make up ordinary substances have all their negative charge electrons paired with positive charge protons. When a stable molecule with paired electrons gains or loses one electron, it becomes unstable. This is called a free radical. Free radicals attempt to stabilize themselves by stealing an electron from a surrounding compound or molecule. When this occurs, a new free radical forms in its place. In turn, the newly formed radical then looks to return to its stable ground state by stealing an electron from another cellular structure or molecule. The chain reaction continues and can occur thousands of times.

Environmental pollution such as tobacco smoke, automobile exhaust and industrial chemicals generate free radicals in our body. Consuming high fat hydrogenated oils like margarine or over-heated fats like French fries, fried meat or fried fish also produce large quantities of free radicals. Some biochemical reactions in the body produce free radicals in small numbers. For example, the production of energy in the cell's mitochondria (the cell's energy factories) or in the production of hormones and in activating enzymes also generate free radical reactions. The immune system also produces free radicals used to destroy bacteria and viruses.

When free radicals are not neutralized they can damage cellular structures. The membrane of a cell contains a fatty acid or lipid membrane, which is less stable than other elements in the body. As a result, free radicals tend to steal electrons at the cell membrane, which initiates a chain reaction known as lipid peroxidation. If this goes unchecked, free radicals can penetrate the cell membrane and damage structures inside the cell including the DNA.

One of the functions of the phospholipid membrane around the cell is to protect the cell from free radical damage. This membrane, made from phosphorous, cholesterol and nitrogen, shields the cell from free radical attacks. Cholesterol in the form of low density lipoprotein (LDL) protects the cell membrane by donating electrons in order to neutralize the free radicals before they damage the cell. The LDL then becomes unstable (rancid or oxidized). This is what gives LDL the term "bad cholesterol." LDL is a critical component of the cell membrane but becomes "bad" when it has been oxidized by free radicals. It is HDL cholesterol (high density lipoprotein) that carries the oxidized LDL cholesterol back to the liver for recycling. Thus, "good cholesterol" helps to clear the 'bad' cholesterol out of the system. However, if the liver is not performing properly or if the bloodstream is clogged with toxins, or if there is too much cholesterol in the bloodstream due to a high animal fat diet, the HDL cannot properly escort the LDL back to the liver. The breakdown in this recycling creates an imbalance in HDL/LDL ratios, leaving the cell exposed to free radical damage. This is because the oxidized cholesterol is not carried away and replaced fast enough to keep up with the free radical attacks to the cell membrane.

Unchecked free radical damage destroys cells and leads to tissue inflammation. This happens when free radicals attack the cells lining our arteries causing tissue inflammation leading to a thinning of the arterial walls. The inflammatory response causes a build up of cholesterol leading to cardiovascular disease.

Dr. Ray Strand, MD, in his book, *What Your Doctor Doesn't Know About Nutritional Medicine May Be Killing You*, details how monocytes (immune cells) gobble up rancid cholesterol, but cause oxidative damage to the endothelium lining of our arteries. It is inflammation from oxidized LDL cholesterol, stuffed monocytes (foam cells) and homocysteine that are the real culprits behind cardiovascular disease.

Homocysteine is an intermediate by-product that occurs when the body is trying to break down the amino acid methionine that we take in when we consume large quantities of meat, milk, cheese, eggs, white flour, and other heavy protein foods that we love. The body uses methylation or re-methylation to regenerate homocysteine back to methionine. In order to perform this, the body needs adequate levels of folic acid, niacin, vitamin B6 (or the active form P5P) and vitamin B12.

The other way the body breaks down methionine is through the trans-sulfuration pathway. In this case, the methionine is converted into homocysteine, which is then degraded into the amino acids cysteine and taurine, which are both important nutrients for cardiac health.[12] This method utilizes a lot of vitamin B6 (P5P) and betaine.

Unfortunately, if our liver is compromised due to pH imbalance, toxin exposure or lack of the precursor nutrients, homocysteine is not converted one way or the other and is left to circulate through our system. This has a toxic effect on the linings of the arteries.[13] There is no safe level of homocysteine. It simply is not supposed to be in our system. An elevated level of homocysteine is a significant risk factor for cardiovascular disease and is implicated in non-insulin-dependent diabetes, rheumatoid arthritis, osteoporosis, and neuropsychiatric disorders.[12]

The body uses various substances called "anti"-oxidants to protect itself from free radical, oxidative reactions. An antioxidant is any substance that readily donates electrons without damaging its own structural integrity. Antioxidants, such as melatonin, help shield cells from free radical attacks just as the paint on your car protects it from rust. While we sleep, melatonin levels increase and circulate through our blood, cleaning our cells by scavengering free radicals. In this way, melatonin reduces the possibility that cells will become carcinogenic each night. Melatonin is one of the most important antioxidants.

The chart below shows free radicals attacking the protective phospholipid membrane of the cell. If this protective shield is penetrated because there is not sufficient antioxidant protection, then free radicals can also damage the cell nucleus, the mitochondria energy centers, and DNA. Free radicals can also destroy hormone receptor sites at the cell membrane as well as hormones within the cell, such as melatonin and/or its receptor site.

Free Radicals
Damage Hormone Receptors, DNA and Energy Factories

(adapted from: "Pro-Hormone Nutrition" by P Yanick, Jr., Ph.D., N.D, and V Giampapa, M.D.)

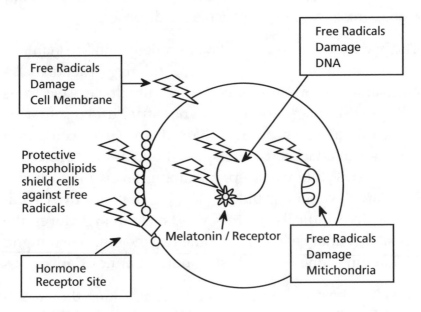

Many antioxidants are found in Nature. For example, lemon juice protects apples from oxidation because the oxygen in the atmosphere steals electrons from the lemon juice first before it starts robbing the apple tissue. An adequate supply of antioxidants is essential for protecting our cells and organs.

When we eat fresh fruits and vegetables we ingest antioxidants like vitamin C found in lemons and oranges and vitamin E found in spinach and avocados. Until recently Nature could provide us with all the antioxidant protection we need. Unfortunately, Nature did not consider that we would create so much pollution that we would have to increase our antioxidant protection. Nature also didn't take into consideration genetically modified fruits and vegetables or that we would over grow our crops and deplete the nutrients in the soil. The result is an ever-increasing need for antioxidants on one side of the equation and fewer antioxidants being provided in our food on the other side. This has created an antioxidant gap.

Optimal physical health today depends on how well we close this gap. Eating organic food is one partial solution to this problem. Studies show that 73 percent of conventionally grown produce had at least one pesticide residue, while only 23 percent of organically grown samples of the same crops contained residues. Therefore, organic food will reduce your exposure to these harmful toxins. However, the term organic is supposed to mean that pesticides are not used on the crops. It is not a guarantee that there are sufficient nutrients in the soil to close the antioxidant gap. If we rely only on the supply of antioxidants we receive from our food, even if it is organic, we will still fall short of closing this gap. For example, because of our nutrient depleted soil we would have to consume 16 oranges each day just to keep up with our increased need for vitamin C.

Vitamin E is one of the most powerful antioxidants for filling the antioxidant gap. It shields the cell membrane from free radical attacks by giving up electrons before free radicals can steal electrons from the cholesterol/phospholipid membrane of the cell. If we protect the cholesterol from oxidation, then we increase our cellular defenses and also avoid the inflammation that free radical damaged (rancid) cholesterol causes to our arteries.

Ensuring that we are getting adequate vitamin E protection is an important first step in reducing cholesterol oxidation. Again, the solution is simple. In order to get adequate vitamin E protection we only need to add 80 organic avocados or 80 organic mangos or 33 heads of organic spinach to our daily meal plan.

Since most of us may have difficulty eating this much in one day, a more practical solution is to add a quality mineral and antioxidant supplement to a diet of organic fresh fruits and vegetables. In fact, the most efficient and practical way to ensure we are closing the antioxidant gap is to take nutritional supplements. If you are suffering from a chronic or degenerative illness it is essential that you close this gap as quickly as possible.

Some of the most important nutritional supplements for cellular health that must be taken every day are as follows:

Vitamin E is one of the most important antioxidants in the human body. It helps to maintain strong cell membranes and protects low-density lipoproteins (LDL) from oxidation.

Carotenoid beta-carotene is the safe provitamin form of vitamin A. Vitamin A promotes healthy skin, a strong immune system, and is important for good vision. In addition, lycopene, lutein, and zeaxanthin are carotenoid antioxidants involved in protecting against free radical damage in the eyes and other organs.

CoEnzyme Q10 (CoQ10) is a potent antioxidant and is essential for energy production in our cells. High levels of CoQ10 are especially important for a strong cardio-vascular system.

Vitamin C is the master water-soluble antioxidant, offering health maintenance throughout the body.

Alpha Lipoic Acid is a vitamin-like antioxidant that is both fat and water-soluble. It is easily absorbed through the intestines and transported across cell membranes. It protects against free radicals, both inside and outside the cell. It is also involved in mitochondrial energy metabolism and recycling oxidized CoQ10.

Grape Seed Extract contains proanthocyanidins (a form of bioflavonoids) that are some of the most powerful free radical scavengers yet discovered. In addition, Grape Seed Extract promotes and maintains sound cardiovascular function by protecting plasma LDL from oxidation.

Garlic contains sulfur-rich derivatives of the amino acid cysteine, which has many health benefits, including inhibition of free radical formation.

Ginko Biloba provides a mix of bioflavonoids that provide antioxidant activity in the brain. It improves oxygenation to the brain and enhances blood circulation throughout the body.

Zinc is a component of hundreds of enzymes related to carbohydrate, fat and protein metabolism. It is also involved in DNA and RNA replication, which is important for healthy cell division and protein synthesis. Zinc functions as an antioxidant and aids in promoting healthy bone structure, immune functions and maintains vision.

Selenium is an essential component of the cell's glutathione peroxidase antioxidant system that neutralizes free radicals created during energy production. It also plays an important role in thyroid hormone metabolism. Selenium is important for prostate health.

Magnesium activates hundreds of enzymes essential to life. It is key to the formation and maintenance of healthy bones and teeth. It also helps metabolize carbohydrates and amino acids and plays an important role in neuromuscular contractions.

Chromium is an important component of the glucose tolerance factor (GTF) that helps to regulate insulin levels and healthy glucose metabolism. Healthy insulin and glucose levels are critical for weight management and for sustained energy levels throughout the day.

Iodine is crucial to thyroid hormone synthesis, which regulates metabolism, growth, reproduction, and protein synthesis.

Copper is essential for enzymes that help synthesize the collagen structures of connective tissue. Copper is also a critical component of the enzyme superoxide dismutase (SOD), an important antioxidant in cell cytoplasm, and it acts as a catalyst in hemoglobin formation.

Manganese is an important co-factor in the production of glycosaminoglycoans, compounds that make up connective tissues, bones, arteries, and other organs.

Manganese also activates numerous enzymes. Supplementation with manganese can enhance the SOD enzyme system to increase antioxidant activity.

Vanadium helps support healthy serum glucose levels and may also support healthy thyroid function.

For hormone support:

Essential Fatty Acids (EFA's) combined with biologically active amino acids are the best approach to enhancing natural hormone production. EFA's are involved in the production of prostaglandins, also known as eicosanoids, that work as hormone helpers in sensitizing cells to hormones, especially sex hormones. They also help control the immune system, the nervous system, the heart, the reproductive system, and the endocrine system. EFA's may help maintain normal blood pressure and healthy levels of triglycerides and serum cholesterol.

Phytoestrogens and Isoflavones are biologically active chemical compounds from grains, legumes, fruit, and vegetables that bind to the same hormone receptor sites as estrogen. This helps stabilize hormonal cycles and may promote long-term reproductive health during and after menopause. It also helps to maintain bone mass. Phytoestrogens protect the body against excess estrogens that are naturally produced in the body or taken in from the environment via pesticides, plastics, and other sources of estrogen-like chemicals that bind to a protein made in the blood. This reduces the amount of aggressive estrogens available to estrogen-sensitive tissue that can be damaged, like the breasts and cervical.

Vitamins B3, B6 and C – along with biotin, magnesium, and zinc – are required to convert EFA's into beneficial prostaglandins type 1 and 3, which help relax blood vessels, lower blood pressure, decrease inflammation, improve nerve and immune function and help insulin work.

For pH support:

Calcium is required for proper bone density. It is found in extracellular fluid and inside the cell where it plays many metabolic roles. It is an electrolyte. It is alkaline. It is critical to normal nerve conduction, muscle contraction, blood clotting, and is essential for producing and activating enzymes and hormones that regulate digestion, energy, and fat metabolism. Calcium must always be taken with Vitamin D (D3 is the active form) for proper absorption.

While all of the above are essential to a high functioning body, taking too many vitamins or the wrong ones in inappropriate ratios may create problems. Taking high dosages of specific and isolated nutrients may be detrimental to your health. Many people have reported increases of their symptoms from taking mega-dosages of many vitamins and minerals.

This is why it is important to know what is in the supplements you are taking and to be sure you are taking quality supplements. Such supplements provide adequate antioxidant protection and nutrition to your cells. There is no sense to buying low quality supplements to save a few dollars only to spend thousands of dollars trying to regain your health down the road. It is better to invest in quality products.

If you are wondering what to look for in a quality product, then you should first consider whether or not the supplement contains all of the antioxidant support required in balanced ratios as well as adequate minerals and vitamin B cofactors. The company should follow Good Manufacturing Practices (GMP) and produce pharmaceutical-grade supplements. This is the only guarantee you have that the ingredients stated on the label are actually inside the bottle. The potency should be guaranteed and you want to know that they are bio-available. In other words, if you are taking a supplement of 100 mg of calcium you want to see the blood serum level of calcium, actually increase after you ingest the product.

Proper cellular nutrition ensures that our cells have the ingredients and energy necessary to perform all of their vital functions. Cells simply do not function properly when they don't have all the nutrients and pre-cursor nutrients to perform their vital metabolic processes and to protect themselves from the damages of free radicals. When our cells are performing at optimal levels we have an abundance of energy. We have vitality. When we combine physical vitality with a positive attitude there is nothing that can prevent us from achieving our highest goals. The right attitude and the right cellular nutrition go hand in hand.

Diet

C ellular nutrition is the result of what we put into our mouths. Supplementation is important. Food is fundamental. What we put into our mouth either contributes to cellular nutrition or depletes cellular nutrition.

Food contains molecular compounds of amino acids, complex carbohydrate chains and various chemical elements, each of which has its own frequency or oscillation. Nutrient vibrations raise body tissue vibrations.[14] Pesticide- and chemical-laden fruits and vegetables, as well as animal protein contaminated with antibiotics and growth hormones, have chaotic vibratory oscillations. When ingested, these foods and substances interrupt the quality of the frequencies we are trying to obtain for our coherent and high vibration nutritional energy needs. If we eat food that causes toxins to accumulate or if it is overly acidic, then our system becomes congested and the flow of nutrients to the cells is restricted. Our food has to be in a pure and coherent energy state because that is what is taken into our cells in the form of biophoton energy and vibration.

Our mental state creates an energy field around us that affects the vibration of the food we are preparing or putting into our mouths. Consequently, if we are dwelling on negative thoughts and feeling while preparing food or eating we are canceling out the beneficial effect of eating high energy food. Our emotions also affect our nervous system. Stress causes the nervous system to activate its sympathetic side. Since the digestive system is controlled and regulated by the parasympathetic nervous system, when we activate the sympathetic nervous system we automatically suppress the parasympathetic nervous system and our ability to properly digest and assimilate our food.

Eating fresh foods and eating light are essential to optimal health. Food that is eaten fresh contains activated enzymes. Fresh fruits and uncooked vegetables with full complements of enzymes are easily digestible and pass through the alimentary tract quickly. Ideally, we should have a bowel movement two to three hours after every meal, not every other day or once a week. It is also important to eat lightly so that there is still the feeling of some rumbling in the stomach, which indicates there are still sufficient gastric juices to digest food. Most people have the habit of eating until they no longer feel this rumbling. They eat until the satiation centers in the brain go on full emergency alert and the stomach feels as though it is about to burst.

There are many cases of people having spontaneous remission of cancer after going on living, uncooked food diets, juicing programs and fasting. Reduced diets take the load off the digestive organs, particularly the liver. The organs of elimination don't have to work so hard. The body's supply of enzymes can be used for clearing foreign protein substances and tumors from the connective tissue rather than for digestion. With the overall energy requirements for digestion dramatically reduced, the body can activate its own healing mechanisms.

Complex Versus Simple Carbohydrates

A carbohydrate is made up of carbon, hydrogen, water and the energy of the sun that plants use to force these elements together. The result is a complex sugar, that when combined with oxygen in the cell, produces the body's energy. Nature provides us with complex carbohydrates in the form of fruits and vegetables.

Naturally occurring carbohydrates are referred to as complex carbohydrates because they are made up of a complex chain that is broken off one at a time by the digestive enzymes so they reach the bloodstream over a period of time. When natural sugar is taken as fruits and vegetables (complex carbohydrates), we also take in other needed nutrients—such as protein, fat, vitamins and minerals—along with the enzymes needed for their digestion.

Simple carbohydrates, in the form of processed food, refined sugar, French fries, potato chips, white bread, cookies, donuts, etc., all lack life-giving enzymes, minerals, and vitamins. Their sugar content is rapidly taken up into the blood stream, causing a high release of insulin needed to normalize the spike in the blood sugar. The insulin reduces the sugar in the blood too far. This puts the body into a panic, provoking an "alarm," or an emergency "survival" response. When the body senses danger, the adrenal glands release cortisol and adrenaline to bring up the blood sugar (glucose) levels. This causes us to go into a sympathetic nervous system overdrive, which consequently suppresses the parasympathetic nervous system. It is the parasympathetic side of the nervous system that runs the digestive system. Over stimulation of the sympathetic nervous system causes blood and energy to be moved away from digestive processes and into processes related survival—increased heart rate, muscle metabolism, etc.

When we constantly eat alarm-triggering food, our digestive system is always under-performing, leading to poor food breakdown and poor nutrient absorption. The undigested food particles putrefy and the related toxins are absorbed by the liver. The liver eventually becomes overburdened and is not able to adequately perform tasks that lead to hormone production, and immune system support. This can lead to gastritis, arthritis, infections, inflammation, degenerative diseases and premature aging.

When we eat complex carbohydrates from fruits and vegetables the sugar content is taken up in a slow and steady fashion and we avoid the above emergency response. A diet of fruits and vegetables also increases our alkaline reserves. If we are deficient in alkaline mineral reserves and we continue to eat a diet that is predominately acidic we will never change the balance. If we eat a diet that is 50 percent alkaline and 50 percent acidic the alkaline balance will stay the same. It is only when we consume more alkaline forming foods than acid forming foods that we start to increase our alkaline reserves. Ideally, we should eat a diet that is at least 80 percent alkaline. Refined sugar, coffee,

The Alarm Reaction from Simple Carbohydrates and Sugars
(adapted from "Pro-Hormone Nutrition" by P.Yanick, Jr., Ph.D., and V. Giampapa, M.D.)

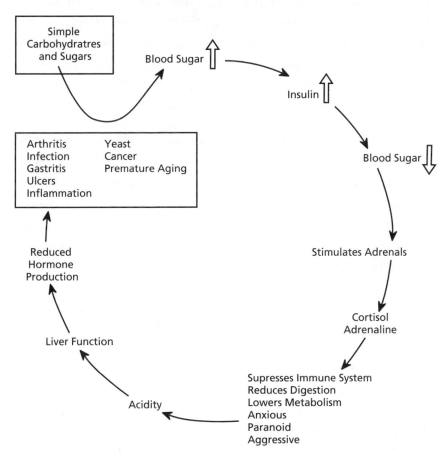

alcohol and animal protein are all acidic or acidic promoting. The ideal diet should be approximately 70 percent raw fruits and vegetables, 20 percent grains and legumes and 10 percent nuts and seeds. Even with this diet it can take three months or longer before the alkaline reserves begin to be adequately replenished.

Most people struggle with this diet in the beginning because they are not used to it. In time, however, they find that they have increased energy and can't imagine eating anything else. If you are not able to follow this diet 100 percent, then by all means make sure you take a quality supplement. This helps to offset the toxicity of your 'normal' diet and to ensure that you are obtaining the nutrients your cells need.

The information given below on some of your favorite food items is not meant to depress you. The information is meant to help you be aware! Be patient. Don't take away all your family's favorite foods at once. The most important thing is to have knowledge. Knowledge is what allows you to make intelligent decisions about what you put in your mouth and what you feed your family.

Protein

Amino acid complexes make up the protein building blocks that give our body structure. There are eight essential amino acids that the body must receive through diet. The other amino acids can be manufactured by the body to produce the various protein structures that are needed. The latter are known as the non-essential amino acids.

There are many myths about how much protein our body needs to stay healthy. The animal-products industry suggests that we need a thirty-percent protein diet. It is important for us to remember that the body's fuel comes from carbohydrates. The body does not use protein as fuel unless there is a deficiency of carbohydrates. Human babies double their birth weight in only six months. Yet, they receive only 2.5 to 3 percent protein when breastfed—the ideal way to feed a baby for the first two years of its life.

Thirty-five grams of protein each day gives a body all it needs to function optimally without undue stress.[15] This is equivalent to 1 cup of quinoa, 1 cup of green beans, 1 cup of broccoli, and 1 cup of peas. A cup of almonds provides 10 grams of protein and 1/3 cup of lentils provides 20 grams of protein. Moderate servings of lentils and some brown rice along with all the fruits and raw vegetables you can eat provides sufficient protein. We can have optimum physical health by eating an alkaline, hormone-enhancing, enzyme and antioxidant rich vegetarian diet.

Consuming excess protein is potentially health-destroying. It congests our cells and forces the pH of our life-sustaining fluids down to cell-stifling, disease-producing levels. Cells overburdened with protein become toxic. Protein eaten in excess of the actual need cannot be properly digested or utilized. Rather, it acts as a poison and carcinogen in the body.

Protein is actually a negative energy food because the body has to come up with more energy to digest protein than the protein itself provides. The rush of energy we get when we eat protein comes from our adrenals, in the same way that we feel artificially energized when we drink caffeine or consume sugar.

Animal protein in particular, is problematic. When animal protein is lodged in the small and large intestines it can remain in the intestines for long periods of time, creating unhealthy bacteria and toxins. We all know what happens to meat when it is left out in the sun. It doesn't take much imagination to picture what putrefying meat looks like sitting in our warm intestines for days or even months.

Pork consumption is a particular problem. If you find that you cannot break the habit of meat consumption, you would be wise to at least avoid pork. The flesh of pigs is used surgically in skin grafts because the skin is particularly compatible with human skin. Pigs eat garbage and consume all sorts of toxins that end up inside their flesh. When we consume their meat we are also consuming the toxins it contains. Since our body does not see this meat as foreign to our own, it readily assimilates it, toxins and all.

Studies have shown that a vegetarian diet provides everything we need to be free of many age-associated diseases.[11, 16, 17] Most vegetables contain much more than 3 percent protein and we assimilate more protein from plants than from animal sources without depleting the energy from our digestive tract.

Sugar

When you eat refined sugar it goes rapidly to the blood. When there is excess sugar in the blood the liver uses it to make neutral fats called triglycerides. Excess triglycerides are stored in the body as fat and also increase blood fats, which can raise blood pressure. The resulting increase in blood fats suppresses the immune system, inactivates macrophages, and can increase infection rates in diabetics. High blood serum fatty acids depress the oxygen transport system. A lack of oxygen at the cellular level interferes with the cell's ability to produce energy. All metabolic processes depend on cellular energy. When cell's become energetically inert and stagnant many degenerative diseases begin to manifest.

Refined sugar consumption also causes deficiencies in B vitamins, chromium, copper and molybdenum. Sugar is responsible for increasing the risk of certain cancers, especially of the breast and colon. Constant high intake of refined dietary sugar over-stimulates or "burns out" normal, healthy pancreas and adrenal functions. Subnormal performance of these two important endocrine glands leads directly to adult-onset diabetes, cardiovascular complications, hypoglycemia, and chronic fatigue. Another direct result of sugar intake is a significant increase in blood serum saturated fatty acids.

Eating refined sugars (in cakes, candies, soft drinks, etc.) also feeds harmful intestinal and vaginal yeast, fungi, toxic organisms, and all forms of cancer. Since sugar and Vitamin C utilize the same transport system, but not at the same time, sugar can prevent Vitamin C from reaching the tissues where it is needed to control or eradicate viruses, fungi, or cancerous organisms that feast on sugar. If this occurs, these pathogens multiply exponentially.

However, never choose aspartame or other artificial sweeteners—they are toxic! Any product with a label stating "Sugar Free" will most likely contain aspartame. The wood alcohol in aspartame rapidly turns into the dangerous carcinogenic formaldehyde in the body. The body converts formaldehyde into formic acid, which in turn causes metabolic acidosis. Aspartame is a neurotoxin that mimics symptoms of multiple sclerosis and other neurological conditions.

The herb 'Stevia' is a safe sweetener substitute. Stevia is naturally very sweet and helps in the metabolism of sugar and is ideal for diabetics.

Oils and Fats

Avoiding fats that cause massive free radical production is a crucial factor in the prevention and treatment of cancer and all degenerative diseases. These fats include: animal fats, margarine, and polyunsaturated cooking and salad oils—such as safflower, sunflower, corn, cottonseed, soy, and others. The best quality oils are contained in fresh whole foods. Nuts and oil-rich seeds are a good source of beneficial oils. They need to be used carefully, however, because of their high oil and protein content. Those with cancer generally do better without foods rich in oil, fat or protein. If cancer patients crave nuts, only the almond has some value, and only if eaten in moderation— a safe limit is usually six almonds daily (must be pre-soaked). Those with cancer must avoid peanuts because they often con-tain the carcinogenic compound aflotoxin and they also retard general metabolism.

There are several major exceptions among oil-bearing seeds. One of the most important is flaxseed because of its immune-enhancing omega-3 content. Flaxseed is also one of the best sources of vegetable lignins; these compounds have antitumor, anti-estrogenic, and antioxidant proper-ties. Flaxseed oil is often used in treating cancer, particu-larly colon and breast cancers, because the cells of these cancers have estrogen receptors that can be inhibited by the anti-estrogenic compounds in lignins. A daily dose of 2 tablespoons is recommended.

It is best to avoid heating oils. When fats and oils are over-heated carcinogenic chemicals known as heterocyclic amines are created. Grilled meat, fried potatoes and broiled fish all contain heterocyclic amines. These hetero-cyclic amines cause cancer by generating DNA-damaging free radicals. One of the best antioxidants used to help stop this damage is found in chlorophyll (fresh, raw green veg-etables). Saturated animal fats, hydrogenated fats like margarine and excessive protein also place a burden on liver metabolism. These fats are often not completely bro-ken down. As a result, partially digested substances enter the bloodstream and can cause abnormal formations such as cancer, especially in previously weakened or injured areas. Animal fat contains arachidonic acid which trans-forms into prostaglandin PGE2 in the body. This substance stimulates cell division, and in excess, may encourage can-cer growth (unchecked cell proliferation). PGE2 can be countered with oils rich in omega-3 and GLA fatty acids (organic flaxseed, evening primrose, and coconut oil).

Dairy Products

Humans are the only animals that drink other animal's milk. Humans are also the only animals to drink milk beyond infant breast-feeding. The consumption of cow's milk is strongly discouraged in infants before they are at least six months old due to the fact that their digestive and immune systems are not mature enough to deal with the complex and large casein milk protein. Cow's milk was meant for 200-pound baby cows, not eight-pound human infants. The result is that young children often develop an allergic response to these large milk proteins. Researchers suspect that the body produces antibodies against these large proteins during infancy. Unfortunately, these large milk proteins are virtually identical to protein in the pancreas. This can cause an autoimmune reaction where the immune system attacks cow's milk proteins and also destroys pancreatic cells, giving rise to child-onset diabetes.

Cow's milk contains a powerful growth hormone that resembles insulin called insulin-like growth factor (IGF-1). This growth factor was intended by nature to promote the growth of a cow by stimulating cell growth. The problem was amplified when the genetically engineered bovine growth hormone (BGH) was given to dairy cows to increase their milk production. BGH increases the levels of IGF-1, which is concentrated in the cow's milk. IGF-1 survives pasteurization and digestion and is absorbed into the blood, where it produces potent growth promoting effects believed to transform normal human breast tissue into cancerous cells.

Some people insist that drinking milk is important for ensuring that they and their children obtain all the calcium they need. Unfortunately, the body may not be able to assimilate calcium from pasteurized, homogenized milk.[10] The high protein content causes milk to be acidic, so the body must pull pH-buffering minerals (calcium) from its bones in order to neutralize the imbalance in the digestive system.

Nature has provided good examples of how we can obtain wholesome nutrition. Cows, horses and elephants all have strong bones provided by the ample protein and micronutrients they ingest by eating plant foods and drinking water. These animals are some of the strongest mammals on earth. And, they seem to have never ending supplies of stamina and endurance.

Caffeine

Caffeine is the most commonly used drug in North America. Caffeine stimulates the brain and artificially and chemically lessens fatigue. Yet, ten (10) grams of caffeine accumulated suddenly in a human body would result in death. Caffeine causes the liver and kidneys to work over-time to rid the body of it. Continuous use of caffeine devitalizes the body to the point where the adrenal glands become so over-stimulated that it takes a high level of caffeine just to feel normal. Caffeine causes the stomach to become more acidic, leading to ulcers of the stomach and duodenum and reduced pancreas function. It can also lead to an overgrowth of harmful intestinal fungi (gut dysbiosis). Caffeine causes the heart to beat faster, the lungs to work harder and the blood vessels leading to the brain to narrow, while increasing the body's metabolic rate. In addition, studies show that caffeine consumption is related to increased bladder and stomach cancers, elevated blood pressure, aggravated diabetes, and may be linked to male infertility as well as birth defects.[18] Caffeine is diuretic and depletes the body of water, pH-balancing minerals and other vital nutrients.

Coffee has a very acidic pH affect and furnishes no

vitamins, minerals, enzymes or protein in the diet.[18] When coffee is roasted, the carcinogen 3,4 benzopyrene is formed. Two other possible carcinogens are found in coffee. Coffee is best avoided if your goal is to achieve optimal physical health.

Pesticides, Food Additives and Genetically Engineered Food

Pesticides, food additives and genetically engineered food are examples of potentially harmful unnatural substances. Unfortunately, they are commonplace as our modernized food industry has made it difficult to avoid them.

The inorganic fruits and vegetables that the average person eats in a year have been sprayed with up to a gallon of pesticides.[15] Pesticides are used by the farming industry to reduce the loss of crops due to infestation. However, these same insecticides and pesticides are also carcinogenic, mutagenic, and toxic to the brain and nervous system. Pesticide exposure is associated with depression, memory decline, mood destabilization and Parkinson's disease.[15]

Food additives such as coloring, preservatives, and flavor enhancers (monosodium glutamate—MSG) are not much better for you than pesticides. Some food colorings have been associated with allergic reactions and hyperactivity in sensitive children. Thirty percent of the population experiences some adverse reaction to MSG at dosages available in food products.[19]

Glutamic acid, from which MSG is derived, is an excitotoxic amino acid as it is known to excite and even kill brain cells in laboratory animals. The following is a partial list of the names in which MSG has been concealed in order to be included in food without being disclosed on the label:

- Monosodium glutamate (MSG)

- Calcium caseinate

- Sodium caseinate

- Textured protein

- Natural flavoring

- Yeast food

- Autolyzed yeast

- Hydrolyzed protein

- Hydrolyzed vegetable protein

- Yeast extract

- Natural chicken or turkey flavoring

- Modified food starch

- Other spices

In sufficient quantities glutamic acid is toxic. To those who cannot metabolize it effectively, even small doses act like a poison. Some common symptoms related to glutamic acid are: anxiety attacks, asthma-like symptoms, attention deficit syndrome, bloating, burning sensations, carpal tunnel syndrome, chest pains, depression, diarrhea, disorientation and confusion, dizziness, drowsiness, fatigue, flushing, gastric distress, headaches and migraines, hyperactivity in children, infertility and other endocrine problems, insomnia, irregular or rapid heart beat, joint pain, mood swings, mouth lesions, nausea and vomiting, numbness of the finger tips, seizures, shortness of breath, simple skin rash, slurred speech, stomach aches, tremors, and weakness.[19]

Pesticides and food additives pose some obvious health threats. What is not so obvious is the issue of genetically modified foods. Foods that are altered through genetic engineering often contain proteins and other components that have never before been part of our diet. These foods are engineered to grow bigger and ripen faster. Some contain their own pest repellents. Some of these genetically altered foods contain proteins from bacteria and viruses. The problem with these foods is that we don't know how our body will react to the foreign, never-before-seen proteins in them. Genetic engineering can give rise to unanticipated allergens and toxins. Genetically engineered foods could be a disaster of untold magnitude. There has been little or insufficient testing to prove their long-term effects.

Sixty to seventy percent of the foods on grocery shelves contain genetically engineered components. They are not subjected to rigorous pre-market safety testing and except for some organic foods THEY ARE NOT LABELED.

Genetically modified foods that have been approved or are awaiting approval or are under development in the USA include:

Apples	Rice
Barley	Soybeans
Beans	Squash
Chestnuts	Strawberries
Corn	Sugar cane
Cucumbers	Sunflowers
Lettuce	Tomatoes
Melons	Tobacco
Peppers	Walnuts
Papayas	Watermelons
Potatoes	Wheat

As previously mentioned, it is extremely important to ensure that the body receives supplementation of the essential vitamins and minerals, carotenoids, bioflavonoids, and other phytochemicals and antioxidants in balanced proportions and at levels high enough to drive metabolic functions and adequately provide protection against the daily bombardment of free radicals.

In addition to taking a daily antioxidant, mineral and vitamin supplement as discussed in the previous chapter, you should also eat a diet containing most, or at least some, of the foods on the list below. We recommend that you buy only organic fruits and vegetables because these foods are grown without the use of pesticides and herbicides, and are not genetically engineered.

Foods to Improve Health

All foods listed are intended to be eaten only in their natural state: organic, unprocessed and unrefined unless noted.

Acorn squash

Alfalfa sprouts

Almonds (raw) fresh,
pre-soaked and peeled

Apples

Apricot kernels

Artichoke

Asparagus

Avocados

Baking powder
(with no aluminum only)
Baking soda

Bamboo shoots

Barley

Basil bay
Beets

Bok choy

Broccoli

Brussels sprouts

Buckwheat whole grain

Burdock

Butternut squash

Cabbage

Lentils

Lettuce

Milk— raw goat
(only in limited amts)

Millet (whole grain)

Mint

Miso (limited amts only)

Mustard greens

Nopales (cactus)

Oat
Oatmeal (also oatmeal
flower)

Oils (flax seed, olive)

Okra

Leaf beans (sprouted only)
Onions

Oregano

Papaya

Parsley

Parsnip

Peppermint

Peppers

Pumpkin

Carrot tops

Carrots (limited amount only)

Cauliflower
Chard

Chayote squash

Cheese
(raw goat cheese—lmt'd amt)

Chicory

Chinese cabbage
Chives

Cilantro

Collard greens

Coriander

Couscous

Cucumbers

Daikon radish

Dandelion root

Dulse

Endive
Fennel

Fenugreek

Flax seed oil

Flour— whole grain

Garlic
Ginger

Ginseng

Green Beans

Pumpkin seeds

Radish

Rice (whole grain brown rice
only)

Rosemary

Rutabaga

Sage

Salt—sea salt only

Scallions
Sea Vegetables

Sesame seeds raw or toasted

Soy products (non-GMO)

Spearmint

Spinach

Sprouts

Squash

Sunflower seeds

Sweetener (stevia)

Tamari soy sauce
(limited amts only)

Tarragon

Thyme

Tofu (non GMO)

Tomatoes—(cooked
only)

Turnip

Turnip greens

Green leafy vegetables

Hazelnut

Jerusalem hearts

Kale

Kelp

Leeks

Lemons

Water

(spring water or
distilled only)

Watercress

Zucchini

Fruit—especially:

Apples

Oranges

Bananas

Blue berries

Mango (alone in am)

Papaya (alone in am)

Pineapple

Foods to Avoid in Order to Regain or Maintain Health

Alcoholic beverages

Baking powder

(with aluminum)

Beef

Beef products

Cheese

(except 'maybe' goat &
tofu cheese)

Chicken

Chocolate

Milk (use only goat
milk—nothing from cows)

Molasses

Oils (use virgin olive oil
only or ghee)

Olives

Pork

Poultry

Processed, refined
foods

Coffee

Corn syrup

Fish

Honey

Margarine

Mayonnaise

Salt (use only sea salt if needed)

Shellfish—(no shellfish at all)

Sodas

Sugar—no sugar of any kind

Vinegar (acidic)

Things to Avoid

- Food Coloring

- Food Additives

- Preservatives

- Pesticides

- MSG or other free glutamates

- Genetically engineered foods

- Hormones from milk and meat

- Sugar

- Caffeine

- Bad fats and oils

- Overheated fats and oils

- Anything cooked in a microwave oven

- Aluminum cooking ware

Some Other "Don'ts"

• Avoid mixing fruit and vegetables together in the same meal.

• Avoid swallowing your food until you have chewed it into liquid in your mouth.

• Avoid frying foods (Bake or cook on the stove instead).

• Avoid eating more than 2 slices of natural, brown, whole grain (not enriched) wheat, kamut or spelt bread per day.

• Avoid eating late at night (try to stop eating by 6 or 7pm).

Sympathetic Dominant Metabolism

Most people have a balanced metabolism and will do well with the recommendations provided above. However, due to genetic constitution or how we respond to stress, our autonomic nervous system can become stuck in the alert mode or in sympathetic nervous system dominance. As we discussed earlier, the alarm response is antagonistic to the parasympathetic nervous system, which controls our digestion. The alarm response also acts to lower our metabolism. Genetics or our response to stress can put us in a state of a lowered metabolic rate. To compensate, we may find ourselves craving foods that help to speed up our metabolism. Simple carbohydrates such as bread, donuts, sweets and caffeine all act to speed up the metabolism and provide a temporary boost that makes us feel artificially energized. Eating protein will act to slow down an already lowered metabolism and therefore, should be avoided. If a slow metabolism is due to stress or toxicity the root cause must be addressed. If one has a genetic tendency towards a slower metabolism then the diet recommended earlier can be adjusted to include more complex carbohydrates and slightly less protein and fats.

Those that are genetically disposed to sympathetic dominance tend to have an excess of cold and dampness in the body creating water retention, sinus problems or bronchitis. In order to bring about a balance the diet should consist of warm, hot and dry foods. It is advisable to eat smaller and fewer meals and to use herbs like ginger, black pepper, cloves, and cinnamon to improve metabolism. Bitter herbs such as aloe, turmeric, and barberry are helpful in reducing sugar and fat cravings. Fruit generally increases mucus and depresses digestion with its high sugar content. For sympathetic dominant types it is best to refrain from eating fruit except for lemons, limes, grapefruit, and limited amounts of cranberries, apples or dried fruits. Vegetables are easiest on the digestion when they are steamed. It is best for sympathetic dominant types to eat chilies, broccoli, cabbage and celery. Other vegetables that are beneficial for those with a slow metabolism are carrots, green beans, fresh peas, beets, asparagus, lettuce, cilantro, watercress, mustard greens, alfalfa, sunflower sprouts, chard, peppers, cauliflower, parsley and spinach. Grains tend to be higher in protein and should be limited to barley, quinoa, corn, millet, rye or buckwheat. Yeasted breads are best avoided. Nuts and seeds are also high in protein and should be eaten in small quantities. Sunflower seeds and pumpkin seeds are best for sympathetic dominant constitutions. Oils should also be used in moderation as they are difficult to digest when the metabolism is slow. Sunflower and mustard oils are recommended. Dairy should also be limited as it tends to be mucus forming. Buttermilk, soy milk and goat's milk are suggested in small quantities.[20]

Parasympathetic Dominant Metabolism

Some people have the constitution of being parasympathetic dominant, where their metabolism is slightly faster than normal. A person with a fast metabolism tends to be thin, never seems to be full, can tend to be anxious, and is a light sleeper. These people tend to do better when they add more protein to the basic diet. Protein, oils and fats require more energy in order to be metabolized and therefore help to satisfy and strengthen the person with a fast metabolism.

Those disposed to a parasympathetic dominant metabolism tend to have cold and dryness in the body. They do better by balancing their diet with foods that provide moisture. Vegetables should be steamed and eaten with whole grains such as wheat, rice, oats, and khus khus. It is best to avoid yeasted bread as it is hard to digest and dry grains like granola and chips. Mung beans are a good source of complete protein. Most other beans cause gas for those with fast metabolisms. Almonds (soaked and peeled), walnuts, pecans, pine nuts, sesame seeds are also good sources of protein. Parasympathetic types do well with oils such as sesame seed oil and ghee. Almond oil, olive oil, avocados and butter are also recommended. Dairy can be beneficial but can also be hard to digest for some. Yogurt, kefir, cream, sour cream, cottage cheese and small amounts of regular cheese can be beneficial for those

with a fast metabolism.[20] Dairy is best avoided for those
that are chronically ill.

Balanced Metabolism

If your metabolism is balanced you tend to have warmth
in the body, you are cheerful, adaptable, and goal oriented.
You do well eating almost anything from the beneficial
food list above in moderation. However, if you consume
foods in excess that are more heat generating, like garlic,
onions or spices, you may experience an imbalance. An
excess of heat affects the small intestines, liver, gallbladder,
spleen, and heart. This can cause you to become hot-tem-
pered, overly critical, impatient and can lead to skin rashes, allergies, eye problems, ulcers, or diarrhea.[20] In order to
bring about a balance you should limit hot and spicy
foods. You will find most fruit to be calming and cooling.
Apples, pears, pineapples, melons, prunes, dates, and
mangos are beneficial for balanced metabolism types. Sour
fruits tend to be too cooling so limit the consumption of
lemons, limes, cherries and strawberries. Most vegetables
are good eaten raw or slightly steamed. It is best for your
type to limit root vegetables like carrots or beets and the
nightshade vegetables (eggplant, tomato, potato) as these
may cause digestion problems.[20] Most grains are balancing
for this type except buckwheat, corn and rye may be too
heat producing.

Metabolism Self-Test

Below is a very simple self-test you can use to determine
your metabolic constitution or tendency. Circle all of the
items under each column that best describes your general
attributes for the most part of your life, not just how you

are feeling in the past few weeks or months. Add up the number of items circled under each column and write the total at the bottom.

Metabolism Self-Test

	Sympathetic Dominant	Balanced	Parasympathetic Dominant
Skeletal Frame	Large	Medium	Thin
Finger Nails	Thick or white	Medium, pink or soft	Thin or cracking
Pulse	60-70 /min	70-80 /min.	80-100 /min.
Weight	Gain easily	Medium or muscular	Low or bony
Stools	Moderate or solid	Loose or burns	Small, hard or gas
Bowel Function	Regular, once a day, sluggish at times	Regular, two times per day	Diarrhea or constipation
Forehead Size	Large	Medium	Small
Appetite	Constant or low, eats slow	Moderate	Strong or excessive, eats quickly
Eyes	Wide, white sclera, long dense eyelashes	Proportional, reddish, light sensitive, yellowish sclera, short eyelashes	Small, dry, itching
Goose Bumps	Often	Occasionally	Rarely if ever
Voice	Slow or silent	High or sharp	Low or weak

Lips	Large or smooth	Medium or soft	Thin dry or cracking
Salt Cravings	Some to none	Moderate	Strong
Speech	Deep and tonal	Moderate or argues	Quick or talkative
Climate Preferred	Warm and mild	Cold and dry	Warm and hot
Sex Drive	Low or steady	Moderate	High, erratic
Menses	Painless with light flow	Moderate cramping with heavy bright red bleeding	Irregular, clots, misses, scanty flow, dark bleeding
Pupil Size	Larger than iris	Same size as iris	Smaller than iris
Sleep	Heavy or deep	Moderate	Light
Temperment	Easy going	Impatient	Nervous or fearful
Memory	Slow to learn but never forgets	Sharp or clear	Quick to grasp ideas but soon forgets
Faith/Beliefs	Constant or loyal	Leader, goal oriented	Radical or changing
Dreams	Few or romantic	Fighting or in color	Flying or anxious
Emotions	Serious, calm, can be greedy or stubborn	Warm, forceful, maybe angry	Enthusiastic, worries, ungrounded
Mental State	Calm or lethargic	Penetrating or critical	Quick or adaptable
Preferences	Water or flowers	Sports or politics	Travel or nature
Total	_____	_____	_____

Some people score high in two categories. This may indicate that you are a combination of both categories or are generally balanced but have a tendency towards one or the other. Every person is different. Please use the above recommendations as a guide. It is best to listen to your own intuition and make changes accordingly and gradually.

Water

The human body is composed of 75 percent water. Brain tissue consists of 85 percent water. Water is involved in the regulation of every process and function of the body. All chemical reactions in the body require water. Hormones and neurotransmitters all rely on adequate solution (water) for transportation and utilization. Water provides structure to the body and increases the efficiency of all protein and enzyme activities. DNA is structurally supported by water and utilizes water pathways to communicate and direct cellular functions and activities. Water is required for all detoxification pathways in the body. The body does not function optimally without adequate levels of hydration. When the body becomes dehydrated it activates the same crisis responses that occur when coping with stress and will begin to mobilize for a "fight or flight" response.[21] Chemicals deployed in the stress response also utilize any water reserves left in the body. Consequently, dehydration causes further dehydration.[21]

Unfortunately, the sensation of "dry-mouth" is not an accurate signal of our body's water needs. In most cases it is the last outward signal of serious dehydration.[21] Seventy-five percent of Americans are chronically dehydrated and with thirty-seven percent of Americans the thirst mechanism is so weak that it is often mistaken for hunger.

Dr. Batmanghelidj, M.D., states in his book, *Your Body's Many Cries For Water*, that water shortages in different areas of the body will cause various signals and symptoms that we now label as diseases. Some important dehydration signals are heartburn, joint and back pain, and headaches. A mere 2 percent drop in body water can trigger fuzzy short-term memory and trouble concentrating. Drinking 5 glasses of water daily decreases the risk of colon cancer by 45 percent, breast cancer by 79 percent and lessens by 50 percent the chances of developing bladder cancer.

A safe rule of thumb is divide your body weight by 2 and use the resultant number to represent how many ounces you should drink of pure water per day. For example, a 170 pound man should drink roughly 85 ounces or 10 glasses of water per day. A 130 pound woman will need to drink 65 ounces or 8 glasses of pure water per day. If you drink caffeinated beverages or alcohol you will need to add at least one more glass of water.

Breath

The oxygen our bodies take from the air is fundamental to our existence because it gives our cells the energy they need to function.

When we inhale, oxygen enters the blood stream. There it combines with hemoglobin to make oxyhemoglobin in the red blood cells and the circulatory system then carries it to the tissues. Cell walls allow the oxygen to pass through and into the cytoplasm (inner cellular fluid), where it finally reaches the mitochondria (small organs or organelles) of the cell. Once in the mitochondria oxygen combines with glucose (natural sugar) to create Adrenosine Triphosphate (ATP). ATP are special chemical molecules that provide short-term stores of energy to the cells. Without a constant production of ATP the cells would stop functioning and we would quickly die.

Like a car, we produce exhaust. When the cell has used or oxidized the glucose, carbon dioxide forms within the cell. Carbon dioxide is a gas that dissolves in the water of our cells to produce carbonic acid. If allowed to accumulate, carbonic acid is poisonous to our cells. Fortunately, it rapidly diffuses out of the cells into the surrounding tissue fluid and back into the capillaries. Once in the blood stream the carbonic acid is partly neutralized by the sodium carbonate present in the blood to produce bicarbonate of soda. When it reaches the lung capillaries, the process is reversed and bicarbonate of soda splits up to produce carbonic acid, which diffuses out of the capillaries into the alveoli as carbon dioxide that is released out of the exhaling lungs. Carbonic acid is poisonous to our cells if allowed to accumulate. If we don't breathe in deeply we also won't breathe out very much. As a result, the carbon dioxide may not be expelled as thoroughly as it should be.

Most of us tend to be shallow breathers. We go through life without paying much attention to our breathing. When we breathe in fully we are providing additional oxygen for our cell's energy requirements. The lungs are also responsible for eliminating most of the acidity that we accumulate in our body. And, this can only happen if we BREATHE. Breathing creates cellular energy on a molecular level (ATP). Breathing removes the acidity that blocks the transportation and utilization of energy throughout the body. Breathing is vital to life.

If you are feeling tired or fatigued or out of energy, consider increasing the volume of your oxygen intake. Do your best to breathe fresh air so you can get plenty of oxygen without any harmful pollutants. If you work in an office building all day and can't open a window, then spend some time outdoors during your lunch break. Sleep with a window open in your bedroom. Get plenty of fresh air and breathe it in as deeply as you can.

Sunshine

If every one on the planet is breathing out carbon dioxide one might think that in time we would all die of carbon dioxide poisoning. Fortunately, green plants take up the carbon dioxide in the atmosphere. They then release oxygen out through a process called photosynthesis. Plants build up sugars and starches on their leaves from the carbon dioxide in the air and from the water taken up by their roots. This combines with the light energy (photons) of the sun to produce oxygen. It is the green matter, chlorophyll that occurs only in plants that allows this reverse respiration to happen.

The sun is not only key to the production of oxygen needed for our existence, it also forces carbon, hydrogen and oxygen together within plants to form complex carbohydrate chains called sugars that provide us with our primary cellular energy source. The sun also provides other important metabolic functions. Sunshine on our bodies helps us to metabolize and better assimilate many needed nutrients. Sunshine on the skin is important in converting cholesterol into vitamin D—an important cancer-fighting vitamin.

When the body first receives sunlight it is split into the prismatic colors, with all their subtle combinations, along with pure white light. The pineal gland is the most sensitive light receptor of the body. The pineal gland is located in a chamber of the brain where it is suspended in cerebrospinal fluid. This makes an excellent point of resonance for the creation of any oscillation or vibration providing part of the overall control of physiological functioning. There are many hormones found within the pineal gland; therefore, this gland is key to the regulation of body rhythms and other regulatory functions as it responds to various frequency oscillations from the sun and the environment.

The pineal gland is known for its production of melatonin, but there are other sunlight sensitive tissues that also produce melatonin such as the retina of the eye and by red blood cells (like the cells of a plant that rely on the sun's energy for photosynthesis). The refraction of the sun's light on the body creates various frequencies or colors that have a stimulating or sedating effect. Everything is vibrating energy and each vibration has its own frequency. Color is a frequency; therefore, every atom or molecule has its own unique color. For example, the prevailing color wave of hydrogen is red, that of oxygen is blue, and each element in turn gives off its own special color.[22]

Viruses and bacteria also emit specific color frequencies as do toxins. We saw earlier that the body receives, stores and emits bio-photon packets of light. It is the frequency information of these photons that provides the regulation and control of all our body processes. These photon frequencies also send out color waves. This knowledge allows us to use color to tune the body into normal balance.

For example, red light has a more stimulating effect on organs and systems, while the color blue is sedative. If we view a burn as the destructive action of the color red (due to the predominance of hydrogen), then it makes sense to treat it by applying the color of oxygen, which is blue. Applying the color blue to a burn victim helps to relieve the strain to the nervous system and to stimulate the healing process.[22]

Activating any part of the body with sunlight or color has many health benefits. Therefore, try to get at least 10 to 15 minutes of sun on your entire body, both front and back daily. (Only 5 minutes on each side if between the hours of 11:00 am and 2:00 pm). This will help stimulate the pineal gland, metabolize and better assimilate many needed nutrients, such as vitamin D. It is best to avoid prolonged exposure to the sun and to avoid sunburns that can damage the skin.

In the simplest of terms, optimal physical health is related to how well we can stay within the amazing cycle Nature intended. Nature's Cycle begins with the sun that provides the energy for plants to generate complex carbohydrates and oxygen that we use for our fuel and respiration. The cycle is completed with our carbon dioxide being transformed back by plants to life supporting oxygen, again, with the aid of sunlight and water. When we stay within this cycle we are providing ourselves with cellular nutrition and maintaining an alkaline pH. This in turn ensures a healthy bio-ecology where cellular and hormonal signaling is effectively transmitted and received and proper bio-regulation and health is maintained.

The challenge is that our life-styles don't necessarily allow us to stick with the program Mother Nature intended. However, if we eat a balanced, healthy, and largely fruit and vegetable diet and combine this with a quality pharmaceutical grade antioxidant, mineral, B-complex supplement along with fresh air, sunlight and pure water, we will have everything our body needs to live to be 100. Our body will have everything it needs for proper self-regulation and self-healing. If we also maintain a positive and hopeful attitude, have faith in ourselves and a sense of inner connection we can also live to be 100 without feeling 100.

Detoxification

A poor diet, exposure to environmental toxins, stress and negative thoughts put us outside Nature's Cycle. Over time, toxins begin to accumulate and disrupt the harmony of our bio-ecology. If our intake of toxins exceeds the liver's ability to eliminate them, eventually the toxins will back up and be deposited in our tissues, joints, and skin. Our ability to eliminate these toxins determines the status of our physical health.

All the stuff that we ingest that isn't good for us has to be broken down and eliminated. It is the job of the liver to break down all these unwanted, unneeded, and even dangerous substances into smaller chemical/molecular units and excrete them through the colon. Metabolic waste from the cells are also carried to the liver to be further broken down and eliminated. This cellular waste is carried away from the cell via the extracellular fluid and is transported to capillaries and lymph vessels within the connective tissue.

The connective tissue is a sponge-like matrix that soaks up toxins and stores them away from vital organs to prevent any damage to them. A heavy onslaught of toxins from a poor diet or environmental pollution is stored in the matrix and then released at a rate that the liver and other detoxifying organs (lungs, kidneys, skin) can handle. This reduces the stress on these organs as well as toxin-sensitive tissues such as the thyroid, pancreas, and nervous system.

When this sponge becomes saturated with toxins, however, it becomes damaged. When this happens the toxins leak out and they become impregnated in the tissues and joints and finally the organs. When the organs become impaired cellular metabolic processes are altered due to an interruption in nutrient supply and waste removal.

Most toxins are first broken down for elimination by a group of enzymes referred to as the Cytochrome P450 enzyme detoxification system or the Phase I detoxification pathway (these are the same enzymes involved in the conversion of pregnenolone into DHEA and other hormones). These enzymes are pH sensitive and will only be activated under a slightly alkaline condition. After toxins are broken down by the Phase I pathway, they are broken down into even smaller molecular units by another set of enzymes known as the Phase II pathway.

Unfortunately, the Phase I process can result in the formation of chemicals that are themselves free radicals. These free radicals can do more damage than the original chemicals from which they were derived. An over activation of Phase I results when we consume substances like alcohol, caffeine, insecticides, benzopyrenes from cigarette smoke and charcoal-broiled meat. Drugs such as codeine, warfarin, phenobarbital, prednisone and steroids, acetaminophen and ibuprofen also activate Phase I.

The free radicals produced by Phase I activity must be neutralized immediately by Phase II enzymes to reduce oxidative damage to healthy cells. This is why cellular nutrition is so important. We must supply the body with the pre-cursor or micro-nutrients needed for the production of these important Phase I and Phase II enzymes.

Some examples of health challenges associated with exposure to environmental toxins and impaired Phase I and Phase II detoxification mechanisms are as follows:[23]

- Autoimmune Disease
- Cardiovascular Disorder Disruption
- Gastrointestinal Disturbance
- Kidney Damage
- Neurological Disease
- Sick Building Syndrome
- Cancer
- Endocrine
- Infertility
- Low Birth Weight
- Obesity
- Spontaneous Abortion

When the sponge-like connective tissue becomes overburdened with toxins it is like a dish-sponge that has become so old that it no longer holds water. When this happens the buffering effect of the matrix is compromised and the liver struggles to keep up. When the liver becomes overburdened with toxins, these toxins begin to spread to other tissues of the body, including the endocrine glands. This affects our hormone regulation and can produce PMS symptoms and exacerbate menopause symptoms.

Estrogen levels are largely controlled by the liver. The body produces three types of estrogen compounds. Estrone (E1) and estradiol (E2) are considered the aggressive types of estrogen because they stimulate cell growth. At high levels they are thought to be associated with increased risk of breast and uterine cancer. Estriol (E3) is the third type of estrogen and is more benign. Estriol contributes to healthy and youthful skin, and may have an anticancer role. It exerts a protective and counterbalancing effect against estrone and estradiol.[24] The liver is responsible for breaking down excess estrogen through a couple of the Phase II detoxification pathways known as methylation and sulfation. When the liver is overburdened this pathway no longer completely breaks down excess estrogen and estrone and estradiol levels can become elevated. Excess estrogen also comes from too much fat in our body, the birth control pill, dairy and meat, chemical spray residues found in our food, estrogen-mimicking molecules (xenoestrogens) from industrial sources—such as plastics, detergents, and synthetic hormone replacement therapy. Estrogen dominance caused by these xenoestrogen excesses blocks the thyroid hormone and leads to uterine fibroids, fibrocystic ovaries and breasts, uterine cancer, breast cancer, other forms of cancers, hypoxia, and edema.[13]

When the body is so toxic that it cannot properly digest or detoxify, it will never derive any benefit from nutrients, and even healthy foods will cause allergic reactions. The best approach to digestive problems, fatigue or any chronic illness is to give the digestive system and the liver a pause/time-out. It is time to relax, quiet the mind and emotions, cleanse, let go and rejuvenate. It may also be time to turn inwardly and examine any negative thoughts or feelings we may be having that are interfering with our digestion as well as any negative behavior that is contributing to our load of toxins. Our physical body often reflects the state of our inward balance.

Reduced Diet

Fasting is a great way to start on the road to optimum health. Since ancient times, people have fasted to train the mind, improve the constitution and treat diseases. Animals fast when they are feeling ill. Today, fasting is used to periodically cleanse the digestive system and to treat a variety of illnesses. Correctly performed, fasting has wonderful effects on such diseases as alimentary disorders, PMS, menopause symptoms, obesity, arteriosclerosis, hypertension, cerebral apoplexy, cancer, heart disease, hepatitis, diabetes, dermatitis, asthma, jaundice, neuritis, epilepsy, and other acute or chronic inflammations. Fasting one or two days during the month can be very invigorating and health promoting.

The reason fasting is so beneficial is that it activates the excretion of noxious waste-matter or toxic substances deposited in the body. It rejuvenates the intestines and eliminates putrefactive bacteria and parasites in the intestines. Furthermore, fasting and reduced diets prevent the stomach and intestine contents from putrefaction and inhibit bacteria toxins from being absorbed into the blood.

Caloric restriction without malnutrition is the only proven method for slowing the human aging process and extending life span.[25] Caloric restriction improves health and well-being because it lowers free radical production in the energy producing mitochondria of the cell.[25] Dietary restriction supports detoxification, increases the levels of antioxidant enzymes and free radical scavengers, and reduces DNA damage and the risk of cancer.[26]

One way of restricting calories is juice fasting. Juice fasting usually consists of a two-week or more program intended to clean out the liver and intestines, while providing cells with a maximum amount of full-potency vitamins, minerals, complex carbohydrates, essential fatty acids, and amino acids to build protein. Fresh juices are packed with digestive enzymes. Because up to 60 percent of enzymatic power is lost within a half-hour of exposure to oxygen, light and temperature changes, it is important to make several batches a day.

The two juices most often recommended are apple and carrot, mixed in a fifty-fifty ratio with distilled water. Apple juice is high in malic acid, pectins, and enzymes that act as a bile solvent and liver stimulant. Carrots are high in beta-carotene, which has a beneficial effect on the liver and on bile flow. Beta-carotene also has been shown to have a significant anti-tumor effect.

In addition, one may add one teaspoon of fiber to the juice four times a day in order to ensure that the small intestine is being cleaned out, along with the colon.

Another way to juice fast is through taking a "green-drink" made from a blend of young barley and wheat grasses, chlorella, brown rice and kelp five times a day.

The nutrients and chlorophyll in this drink build blood, oxygenate cells and act as scavengers of free radicals.

Enemas are always taken while juice fasting in order to help eliminate the toxins that are loosened and expelled from the system. During fasting natural bowel movements stop, leaving toxic wastes in the system. For this reason, those who fast use enemas every day. If you fast without enemas toxins remain in your colon and are re-absorbed directly into the liver where they poison your whole body. Enema formulas made with herbs such as chaparral, yellow dock and wheat grass stimulate the liver and gallbladder to remove toxins, open the bile duct, encourage increased peristaltic action and produce the necessary enzyme activity for healthy red blood cell formation and oxygen uptake.

As a warning, during or after a detoxification protocol you may feel worse. For example, most people undertake a detoxification program without first ensuring that their organs of elimination can handle the down-load of toxins. If, for instance, your gallbladder is blocked or restricted and the liver is not able to pass these toxins through the bile the toxins have no where to go except into the blood. In this case, the kidneys have to eliminate them or the toxins are discharged into the lymphatic system or come out through the skin. Skin rashes, blisters, and other breakouts of the skin may occur for this reason. Other symptoms are headaches, body aches and a general feeling of tiredness or worse. Some refer to this as a "healing crisis." This is not a healing crisis. This is a mistake. It is a common mistake made by over-eager people in their attempt to get the toxins out of their body as fast as possible. In order to avoid these uncomfortable reactions it is important that we balance the pH first so we ensure that all the proper detoxification enzymes are activated and doing their job of breaking down and neutralizing these toxins.

After we have balanced the pH we need to make sure the colon is "open" and functioning properly because the colon is the major exit route for the liver toxins. We have to make sure that the intestines are healthy and able to withstand the flow of toxins. If you are constipated or suffering from intestinal inflammation of the lymph or mucus membrane, or you are suffering from leaky gut syndrome, where food particles pass through the intestinal walls, then you do not have a secure exit route. When this occurs, mobilized toxins cannot be eliminated and instead will create additional inflammation and damage to other organs and tissues as they re-settle. This is why it is critical to heal the intestines first. A good rule of thumb is to ensure you are regularly having two to three bowel movements per day before you start any detoxification program.

The second step is to ensure that the kidneys, lymph system and bile duct are all open and working properly. If not, then these organs and systems must be detoxified, strengthened and supported first before embarking on a general detoxification program. The status of these systems is generally best left to your health care provider. If you suffer from edema or have any urinary problems then chances are these systems will need to be strengthened prior to detoxification.

The skin is a mirror to our health. In fact it is our largest detoxification organ. There are areas of the skin that correspond to various organs. When these organs eliminate toxins through the skin, the skin area corresponding to the organ is affected. Conversely, what we put on the skin also affects the underling organs for better or for worse. If we use natural products on our skin they will support the organ nutritionally. Many cosmetics and cleaning products contain substances that are carcinogenic or toxic to our bodies. Using these products on the skin directly impacts underlying organs. Our kidneys and liver are constantly working to process and detoxify the blood. Toxins from the liver and kidneys are partially eliminated through the skin. Many skin problems and skin diseases are seen over those areas associated with liver and kidneys. When the organs can no longer process toxins efficiently, the skin is called upon to assist.

When the skin is covered with paraffin from body lotions, sunscreen and other cosmetic products, it is like wrapping the skin in plastic. This prevents the skin from helping the organs to eliminate toxins. As a result toxins are reabsorbed into the body where they are stored in the fatty and connective tissue. Some sunscreens contain paraffin and heavy metals that seal off the skin, preventing it from breathing, perspiring, and releasing toxins. The trapped toxins "cook" under the heat of the sun, causing cellular damage that can lead to skin cancer.

In addition, it is best to avoid other un-natural products that can affect the skin or are absorbed through the skin placing a burden on our detoxification mechanisms. Some of these products are permanent wave solutions, hair colors, toxic hair sprays, synthetic cosmetics, lipsticks made out of coal tar dyes, and antiperspirants with aluminum ingredients. Use natural cosmetics. Use only non-allergenic natural deodorants. A fresh lemon cut in half and spread under the arms makes an excellent, long lasting deodorant.

It is important to avoid using toothpaste that contains fluoride. Fluoride and iodine are both members of the halogen group of atoms and have an antagonistic relationship to all other elements. Excess fluoride in the body can interfere with the iodine dependent functioning of the thyroid gland. If in doubt, don't use it.

It is also best to avoid cleaning solutions, solvents, paint removers, and insect sprays. All of these chemicals are toxic to the body and require additional liver detoxification support. If you have a degenerative disease it is advisable to take the extra precaution of removing all toxic cleaners or other toxic items under your sink. Move them into the garage or somewhere far away so you are not breathing their fumes or coming in contact with them in any way.

Eating and cooking utensils should be free of aluminum. It is best to cook with stainless steal or glass. Teflon-coated pots and pans may pose a health risk. The chemical, perfluorooctanoic acid (PFOA) used in manufacturing teflon-cookware, water- and stain-resistant clothing, cosmetics and other products has been linked to testicular, liver and pancreatic cancer in animals.

Rely on the sun to illuminate your room or use full-spectrum lights or candles. Avoid fluorescent lights as much as possible. The insides of fluorescent tubes are filled with mercury vapor. Also, DO NOT USE ELECTRIC BLANKETS. Research has shown increased incidence of cancer with persons using electric blankets. You may heat your bed with an electric blanket, but turn it off prior to getting into bed.

Extra Low Frequencies (ELF's)

Toxins in our food and from the environment are shown to be potentially carcinogenic and place a large burden on our body's ability to detoxify itself of these carcinogens. Evidence is mounting that electromagnetic radiation damages cells in a way that is also potentially cancer causing. Unfortunately, we are not able to counterbalance their effects with normal detoxification mechanisms.

The electromagnetic radiation generated by the 60hz AC current going through your home, cellular phones, domestic appliances, industrial machines, computers, radio and television transmitters, electric shavers, hair dryers, electric blankets, air conditioners, high tension wires, fluorescent lights, and other devices is bombarding us at levels never before experienced by human beings. This electromagnetic radiation may cause psychological effects, such as tension, anxiety, lowered resistance to bacterial and viral infections, and changes in hormone levels, blood sugar, and enzymes. Electromagnetic frequencies disrupt the DNA signaling that regulates and controls all biochemical processes.

Biophysicist Dr. Neil Cherry, a New Zealand-based researcher, who experiments with the hazardous effects of ELF's, shows that electromagnetic radiation from power lines and appliances can reduce the antioxidant protection effect of melatonin on human breast cancer cells. For example, he describes how a laboratory took human breast cancer cells and exposed them to an infusion of melatonin. Then they applied a very low level of varying electric field and the protective effect of melatonin was totally eliminated.

Those who work in the electrical industry are at particular risk. This is because the ELFs act as co-carcinogens preventing cellular repair mechanisms from working. Not only may cancer result, but people may also suffer from depressed immune systems. A panel of three California health scientists concluded that electromagnetic fields from power lines, appliances and wiring in homes and schools can increase the risk of childhood leukemia, adult brain cancer, Lou Gehrig's disease, miscarriages and other diseases.[27]

Those with cancer or other degenerative illnesses are advised to avoid ELF exposure as much as possible. It would be better not to place your bed near an electrical outlet or sleep with a radio or digital clock on your bed stand. Avoid having a television in your bedroom. As much as possible, reduce exposure to appliances that may disrupt cellular signaling and communication.

Stress Management

Stress and how we deal with stressful situations is directly related to cellular degeneration. The "flight or fight" response to a dangerous situation is stressful. However, we can also provoke a "flight or fight" response or "stress response" when experiencing a simple annoyance such as being cut-off in traffic. Chronic stress can arise from everyday living experiences such as dealing with demanding bosses, hurried schedules with children, relationship problems, etc., etc.

During stress the adrenal hormones, adrenaline and cortisol, re-direct resources from various cells throughout the body to provide maximum energy for survival responses to life-threatening situations. This same response happens even when the situation is not life-threatening but we allow it to make us feel angry, overwhelmed or out of control. It is a primitive and instinctual survival response. When it occurs, the hormone adrenaline signals the liver and tissue to release stores of glucose (sugar) to be used for the energy needed to run away or to fight. Adrenaline also directs blood supply toward the heart and lungs in order to improve oxygen and blood supply to muscles. Blood and energy are conversely moved away from digestion processes to save on energy (Nature doesn't expect you to stop for lunch while you are running away from a life-threatening situation). The hormone cortisol kicks in and stops the pancreas from secreting insulin in order to maximize glucose availability in the bloodstream. This is one reason chronic stress can contribute to diabetes. Cortisol also cannibalizes amino acids, the cells' building blocks, in the cells for quick energy. Chronic cannibalism of the body's resources and structures leads to degeneration. Cortisol also inhibits thyroid hormones, which reduces the metabolic energy normally used for digestion and detoxification (liver function).

The metabolic by-products of adrenaline and cortisol are acidic. This contributes to the inactivation of hormones and enzymes required for digestion, detoxification and cellular repair and maintenance. It also causes a loss of electrolytes and a demineralization of bone that can lead to osteoporosis.

In addition to being acidic and contributing to cellular degeneration, cortisol also suppresses the immune system. One of the functions of cortisol is to reduce the inflammatory effect caused by a wound. This speeds up wound healing during a fight for survival. Cortisol's anti-inflammatory effect is caused by its suppression of the immune system. The immune system uses toxic agents that kill invading bacteria at the site of a wound. The immune system agents that kill bacteria are also inflammatory to healthy tissue. Nature figures if you survive the fight you can worry about the bacteria later. However, when we are under constant stress we are also chronically suppressing our immune system, which opens the door to chronic illnesses.

When we are constantly fighting with our partner, boss, co-workers, or just worried about it in our mind, we are living in a state of constant adrenal stress as well as adrenaline and cortisol over-production. Adrenal stress can occur from anger, fear, worry, guilt, and mental or physical strain. It can also be caused by sleep deprivation or going to sleep late, chronic infection, temperature extremes, toxin exposure, and nutritional deficiencies. The long-term effect is that the adrenal glands become impaired. This can lead to such symptoms as low body temperature, lowered output of gastric juices, indigestion, weakness, hair loss, depression, irritability, muscle loss, low blood pressure, dry skin, insomnia, food and inhalant allergies, PMS, craving for sweets, auto-immune diseases, a suppressed immune system and cancer.

If you suffer from chronic stress you may benefit greatly from such tools as Scalar Heart Connection or Holographic Repatterning. These methods can help you change your emotional response to various stressors in your life. When we maintain our balance and composure during stressful situations we keep our adrenal stress response out of the picture. This helps us live longer and healthier. And, we may also find that our balance and composure helps those we love around us who may be going into stress responses themselves because of our anger and stress response.

One of the ways Nature helps us calm down and reset our rushing hormones after a stressful situation is with DHEA. It helps calm the system down after a successful fight or flight. DHEA is the anti-stress hormone because it is antagonistic to cortisol. This means that excess cortisol suppresses the production of DHEA. DHEA, on the other hand, suppresses cortisol and, therefore, can reverse the immune suppression caused by excess cortisol levels. This is beneficial in improving our resistance to bacteria, viruses, parasites, and candida. This is why the DHEA/Cortisol ratio is an important measure of immune function.

The primary gland that responds first to danger or a threatening situation is the pituitary gland. When the pituitary senses danger it releases a hormone that stimulates the adrenal glands to secrete adrenaline and cortisol. The pituitary also secretes various hormones that regulate the production of thyroid hormone and gonadal hormones (estrogen, progesterone, and testosterone). When we are constantly under stress the pituitary gland begins to fatigue and no longer produces all the other various hormones needed for a variety of regulatory processes. For example, a reduction in the pituitary's production of thyroid hormones can reduce cellular metabolism, resulting in insufficient cellular energy needed by the liver for detoxification. Reduced pituitary function can also result in adrenal exhaustion and hypothyroidism as well as reduced levels of sex hormone production. This can result in chronic fatigue, fibromyalgia, arthritis, diabetes, cardiovascular disease, and cancer.

In addition to the Scalar Heart Connection and Holographic Repatterning techniques that help us to resolve inner-conflicts and inherited beliefs that cause us to react to situations in a stressful manner, laughter and breathing are both good ways to reduce stress and to help re-set the over-stimulated sympathetic nervous system. The B vitamins, particularly vitamins B-3 (niacin) and B-5

The Psychological Effects of Stress

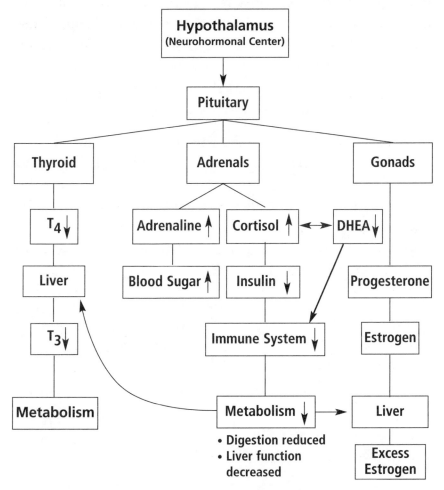

(pantothenic acid) are important anti-stress vitamins. The adrenal glands can be additionally supported with antioxidants, Siberian ginseng, lipoic acid, vitamin B-6 or the active form P5P, and GABA. Recommendations for pituitary gland support include the amino acids arginine, glycine and tyrosine. The thyroid can be supported with the herbs bladderwrack, alfalfa, and yellow dock root.

Our Grandmother's advice to just laugh our troubles away is becoming scientifically recognized as sound advice. Laughter produces endorphins that provide feelings of joy and relaxation that can relieve pain and alleviate stress. Not all of us are used to laughing, however. We are so full of stress that we forget to take time out to laugh and enjoy ourselves or those who are dear to us.

Physiologically, when we laugh we dispel carbon dioxide and replace it with oxygen-rich air, providing physical and mental freshness. Laughing can produce anti-inflammatory agents that can aid back pain and arthritis. It encourages muscles to relax, and exercises muscles all over the body. It also reduces the levels of cortisol, which is responsible for immune suppression.

According to Dr. Lee S. Berk from Loma Linda University, California, USA, laughter helps to increase the count of natural killer cells (NK cells—a type of white cell) and also raises antibody levels. Researchers have found that after laughter therapy, there is an increase in antibodies (Immunoglobulin A) in the mucous of the nose and respiratory passages, and that laughter may provide protection against some viruses, bacteria and other micro organisms.

According to Dr. William Fry of Stanford University, one minute of laughter is equal to 10 minutes on the rowing machine. In other words, laughter stimulates heart and blood circulation in a way that is equivalent to any other standard aerobic exercise. Laughter exercise is suited for sedentary people and those who are confined to a bed or wheelchair.

The physical effects of laughter on the body result from increased breathing, oxygen use and heart rate, which stimulate the circulatory system. Many hospitals and ambulatory care centers have incorporated special rooms where humorous materials, and sometimes people, help make people laugh. Materials commonly used include movies, audio and videotapes, books, games, and puzzles. Many hospitals use volunteer groups who visit patients for the purpose of providing opportunities for laughter.[28]

So, laugh as many times as you can throughout the day. Practice laughing by taking a deep breath and letting it out with a strong but slow Ha!, Ha! Ha! Squeeze in your belly with each Ha. Take another deep breath and again release the Ha! Ha! Ha's, but more quickly. The Ha! Ha! Ha's get faster and faster with each breath, until you, or you and the person you are laughing with, are in a full belly laugh.[8]

Another way to reduce stress is to take some time each day for relaxation. For at least half an hour daily do something which gives you enjoyment and produces peace, calm and contentment for you. This may be a quiet time you spend in your garden, listening to music, swimming, yoga, puttering in your workshop, reading a favorite book—whatever you like doing. The more activities you can involve yourself in which are positive and enjoyable, the faster your recovery will be.

In addition, throughout the day observe your body. Are you tense? Are all your muscles relaxed? How can you change your position to make yourself more comfortable and relaxed?

Movement and Fitness

Do you walk three times per week? Do you go to the gym? Do you practice any kind of movement more than twice a week? Do you practice yoga, stretching, dancing or rope jumping?

Life is energy in motion. Movement is Life. Movement integrates your brain hemispheres. Movement produces endorphins of pleasure that boost your immune system. Movement orients you to yourself, to the environment and to others so you move in the direction of joy and love.[8]

Movement also produces and strengthens electrical fields in the body. Tissues in the body generate electric fields when they are compressed and stretched.[29] With each step we take we are compressing bones, which generates an electrical field. When cartilage is compressed, or when the skin is stretched or bent, a minute electric pulsation results. The body is electric. Movement increases our energy levels by generating bio-electricity.[29]

Movement works to move the lymph throughout the body. The lymphatic system picks up toxins that have been excreted by the cells or have been deposited by the open blood capillary ends. The lymph is a clear, watery, interstitial fluid that is known as 'lymph' when it drains into the network of lymph capillaries. The lymph system contains lymphocytes and other immune system cells that ingest bacteria and debris. The lymphatic fluid is not pumped, but is moved when lymph vessels are compressed by surrounding muscles as they contract during movement. This is why walking, and particularly jumping rope or bouncing on a rebounder (trampoline), are so important.

Get Some Exercise

Each morning, after you have been awake for a short time and have moved about a bit, take 15 minutes to stretch. Depending on your condition, you may or may not be able to stretch your entire body. Stretch as many limbs and joints as you can, slowly and without experiencing pain. There are many books you can obtain to show you simple and effective stretches. Peter Kelder's book, *Ancient Secret of the Fountain of Youth*, explains five Tibetan rites or exercises that are beneficial. Beginning yoga stretches are highly recommended. If you are in pain, you may want to consider visiting a physical therapist to assist you in establishing a routine that is best for you. In addition, always change your position and stretch if you have remained in one position for 15 minutes or longer. Most animals, particularly cats, do this instinctively.

Unfortunately, so many of our jobs or lifestyles do not encourage varied movements so we don't use all the parts of our body throughout the day. Keep your entire body flexible. Stretch and move your toes, legs hips, arms, fingers, neck, spine, etc. Stretch your facial muscles too. Make funny faces. Stretching in a swimming pool is a wonderful way to begin increasing your flexibility, and many people whose bodies are particularly inflexible find stretching in the water the easiest way to begin.

Sleep

As important as movement is for the body the time when we are not moving while asleep allows the body to rest and repair. There are 4 levels of sleep from the light REM (rapid eye movement) stage to deep sleep stage 4, where the restorative process takes place. Studies have shown that those whose sleep was interrupted before falling into stage 4 over a two-week period developed chronic fatigue syndrome symptoms.

One of the most important aspects of deep sleep is the increased secretion of HGH (human growth hormone) and the elimination of free radicals in the brain. Small amounts of HGH are secreted during the day, but the vast amount is released during sleep. HGH stimulates tissue regeneration, liver regeneration, muscle building, breakdown of fat stores, normalization of blood sugar regulation, and many other beneficial processes in the body.

Sleep itself functions as an antioxidant as free radicals are removed from the brain during sleep. Sufficient sleep ensures minimal neuronal damage from free radical accumulation during waking hours. For this reason, chronic sleep depravation accelerates aging of the brain.

Melatonin, as discussed in an earlier chapter, is a hormone manufactured by the pineal gland. Melatonin secretion is stimulated by darkness and is suppressed by light. Melatonin is capable of permeating any cell in any part of the body. It protects the nucleus of the cell against free radical damage to DNA. Melatonin supplementation has been shown to inhibit several types of cancers. Environmental exposure to electromagnetic fields may cause a suppression of melatonin synthesis, which in turn may leave the DNA exposed to free radical damage and provoke carcinogenesis. Patients with chronic progressive multiple sclerosis have lower melatonin levels compared to those with patients whose multiple sclerosis is in remission.[12]

Seven to eight hours sleep is essential for proper regeneration and repair throughout the body. To prepare for restful sleep avoid TV for one hour before bedtime. Do not eat or watch TV in bed (retain the association that "bed" is for sleep). Wind down one hour before bedtime, minimize stimulating noises, activities, food intake, etc. Instead, meditate, take a bath or read something uplifting.

Try to go to sleep before 10 pm, the time when all your hormones are at their highest peak.

The chart below is based on the Chinese Meridian system and shows the time of the day or night where the organ or system is most active and the time where it is least active. Times during the day or night when you feel discomfort may be a signal that the corresponding organ (either high activity or low activity organ) may be stressed. If you always wake up at night check the time you generally wake up to see if you can gain some insight into what system or organ may be under stress. For example, if you wake up every night around 2 am to go to the bathroom or for no reason at all, your liver may be calling for some attention.

Time	High Activity Organ/System	Low Activity Organ/System
7am–9am	Stomach	Heart Protector
9am–11am	Pancreas/Spleen	Triple Warmer (hormones)
11am–1pm	Heart	Gallbladder
1pm–3pm	Small Intestines	Liver
3pm–5pm	Bladder	Lungs
5pm–7pm	Kidney	Large Intestines
7pm–9pm	Heart Protector	Stomach
9pm–11pm	Triple Warmer (hormones)	Pancreas/Spleen
11pm–1am	Gallbladder	Heart
1am–3am	Liver	Small Intestines
3am–5am	Lungs	Bladder
5am–7am	Large Intestines	Kidney

Dental Health

Dental health incorporates many of the principles covered throughout this book. Although people are unaware of the role that dental health plays in our well being, it is absolutely fundamental. While the principles of diet, cellular nutrition, maintaining an alkaline pH as well as stress management are critical in supporting a strong immune system, a weakened immune system allows dental bacteria to flourish. Dental bacteria produce acidic by-products that deplete calcium levels in the blood and can migrate to other areas and organs in the body, and create areas of disease known as focal infections.

Most people are unaware that each individual tooth is energetically connected to various organs and systems in the body, as seen in the summary chart on the following page.

The chart indicates that tooth #6, commonly referred to as an eyetooth, is related energetically to the liver, gallbladder, eyes, posterior pituitary gland, foot, back of the knees, and hips. These relationships are not hard to understand when we consider that all of the organs and systems of our body developed from the same basic embryonic cells. These cells migrated and differentiated during fetal development into specific cells, but maintain an energetic

Tooth/Organ Relationship
(Right Side of Mouth Shown Only)

Endocrine Glands	Pituitary – Ant.	Thyroid	Thymus	Pituitary – Post.	Pineal
Sensory Organs	Ear Tongue	Tongue	Nose	Eye	Nose
Organs	Heart Duodenum Terminal Ileum	Pancreas Stomach	Lung Colon	Liver Gall-bladder Biliary Ducts	Kidney Bladder Rectum
Tissue Systems	Central Nervous				
Other Systems	Mammary Gland				
Upper Teeth	#1	#2/3	#4/5	#6	#7/8
Lower Teeth	#32	#31/30	#29/28	#27	#26/25
Other Systems		Mammary Gland			
Tissue Systems	Peripheral Nerves	Arteries Veins	Lymph		
Organs	Heart Terminal Ileum	Pancreas Colon	Lung Stomach	Liver Gall-bladder Billiary Ducts	Kidney Bladder Rectum
Sensory Organs	Ear Tongue	Nose	Tongue	Eye	Nose
Endocrine Organs				Gonad	Adrenal

resonance or connection with each other that causes a sympathetic reaction, regulation, and compensation.

Dr. Weston Price, a dentist in the 1930's, was one of the first to recognize and document how an infection in a specific tooth can cause degeneration in the associated organ. In one study Dr. Price removed root-canal teeth from patients who had developed heart disease following a root canal procedure, and he found that the patients' heart disease improved. He later implanted the extracted root-canal teeth into healthy rabbits and they immediately developed heart disease and died.[30]

The bacteria stemming from root canals can mutate into more virulent forms as they attempt to adapt to an oxygen-depleted environment. These bacteria can then migrate from the root of the tooth into the bone and cause infections called cavitations. Cavitations are so dangerous because they produce toxic poisons including noxious sulfur compounds and gasses such as mercaptans, thioethers and others.[31]

The toxic by-products of dental bacteria are extremely acidic and rapidly deplete the acid-buffering ionic calcium in the bloodstream. People with degenerative diseases have low levels of ionic calcium. When the offending dental infection is removed, the ionic calcium levels are usually restored. Some people who are vegetarians or who have eaten a primarily alkaline diet for years, yet still have an acidic system (saliva litmus paper reading below 7) discover that they have dental bacteria and/or heavy metal toxicity. Under this condition it is simply impossible to change the pH to a slightly alkaline one. If you find it impossible to change your morning saliva pH to at least 5.8, then you will need to consider the possibility that you have a dental infection or heavy metal toxicity.

Periodontal infections can go undetected for years as the body seals off and encapsulates the pathogens deep within the jaw. The infection produces an energetic imbalance as well as a constant stress on the immune system. Toxic gas, known as dimethylsulfite (CH3-S-CH3), is emitted from these dental infections.[32] Dimethylsulfite causes immune malfunction and can lead to paralysis of the heart and/or coronary infarct.

Dental bacteria and their toxic by-products slowly leak into the bloodstream and make their way to tissue near and far away. Once there, they can cause focal infections in other areas of the body. Circulating bacteria and their toxins place an enormous stress on the immune system as it attempts to keep the infection under control. This may take place for years without any noticeable symptoms. However, when people with this condition suffer an emotional upset such as an accident, a death in the family, or an unpleasant divorce, the immune system is overtaxed. Once the immune system can no longer keep up with the infection, the bacteria begin to multiply and more serious conditions can develop, i.e., rheumatism, arthritis, heart problems, and/or cancer.

Heavy metals found in dental materials are also a source of toxicity and immune suppression. Dental fillings that contain mercury (found in amalgam fillings) as well as gold crowns containing palladium and caps containing nickel can place a toxic burden on the connective tissue and organs. Abnormally high concentrations of these metals in the body will stimulate macrophages and monocytes, the scavengers of the immune system, to engulf these toxins. These scavengers do not possess enzymes capable of breaking down these metals, so they continue to stay within the immune cell. A macrophage that is clogged with metals cannot engulf bacteria and viruses. When these metal-containing cells die, the metals in them return to the general circulation, where they eventually bind to tissue and organelles of the cells, such as mitochondria. When these metals bind to mitochondria, the energy production of the cell is inhibited or blocked. Once this happens, the cell goes into "survival mode" and begins to divide uncontrollably, and carcinogenesis is under way.

When mercury finds its way into the connective tissue it can be picked up by the autonomic nervous system. The autonomic nervous system is connected to every cell in the body. Nerve cells are constantly picking up nutrients and other materials from the ends of their filament-like structures. Nutrients are transported to the cell body via structures in the nerve axons, called microtubules. The microtubules are also responsible for discharging material out of the cell. When the microtubules pick up mercury this metal blocks the formation of tubulin. Tubulin is a protein that must be present in order to form microtubules. If the microtubules are loaded with mercury there is no way for the cell to obtain nutrients, to discharge toxins, or to rebuild itself. The end result is that the cell starves and the axon transport system is shut down. This leads to chronic diseases such as Alzheimer's and multiple sclerosis.

Another problematic toxic metal found in dentistry is palladium. Metallurgy reports have revealed that even some dental gold material (which is supposed to be the most compatible heavy metal with our body) actually contain 17 to 40 percent palladium. Palladium is a highly toxic material (it literally makes holes in your brain). Holistic medical doctors in Germany refer to palladium as the "fool's gold" of dentistry because it may be more dangerous than mercury. Both mercury and palladium bind with the amino acid methionine (S-adenosylmethionine) in the digestive tract and once synthesized, these methylated metals easily diffuse through cell membranes and disrupt enzymatic activity. The affinity these and other metals have to binding to methionine can cause a protein configuration that is detected by lymphocytes as something foreign. Methionine is a major source of numerous sulfur-containing compounds. When metals bind to sulfur derived amino acids in the food we ingest, an adverse immune reaction can occur in the gastrointestinal tract. Food and gluten allergies can result as can certain auto-immune disorders.

Dr. Elef Karkalis, M.D., of Oppenheim, Germany, states that early symptoms of palladium overexposure are chronic fatigue, allergies, headaches, lymph node swelling and immune weakness. More advanced toxicity can give rise to bronchitis, muscle and joint pain, memory loss, digestive and nervous disorders, weight loss, chronic sinusitis and tinnitus, excessive sweating, neuralgia, facial paralysis, depression, sleeping disorders and muscle weakness.

Many bridges have porcelain caps supported by a nickel base. Apart from being carcinogenic, nickel also commonly produces local inflammatory reactions on the skin. It is estimated that about 5 to 13 percent of all cases of eczema are caused by contact with nickel or nickel compounds. Cancer of the lungs, nasal mucosa and the larynx are the most serious consequences of long-term occupational exposure to nickel.

In addition to the toxicity of the metal itself the combination of several different types of metals generates electrical currents. These different metallic fillings act like a battery that generates electrical current through the mouth and head and can be easily detected with specific meters in the milli-volt and milli-amp range. These electrical currents often interfere with the body's own electrical impulses that control a wide variety of functions. The build-up of voltage close to the base of the skull and the hypothalamus can have regulatory consequences to various neurohormonal functions.

The combination of dental bacteria and heavy metals can be lethal. The by-products of the bacteria and the presence of heavy metals are both acid-forming in the bloodstream. This causes micro-bacteria known as mycoplasma in the blood to adapt to the acidification of their environment by mutating into forms that are cancer-provoking. These microorganisms cannot tolerate changes in the pH balance of the blood and tissues. When the tissues become overly acidic there is less oxygen available. This forces mycoplasma to change their metabolism to an anaerobic metabolism. This mutation causes the mycoplasma to become larger and their metabolic by-products to become toxic to healthy cells. In this state they are known as pathogenic

Mycoplasma. Pathogenic mycoplasma are always found in areas of the body where immune defenses are not present. One of the best places to find these mycoplasma is in the platelets, which are the smallest cells in the blood needed for blood clotting. Mycoplasma and viruses use platelets as carriers to travel through the circulation system undetected by immune defenses.[32]

Mycoplasma penetrates cells and causes cellular alterations. It also produces ammonia and oxidized compounds (hydrogen peroxide, peroxide compounds), which are all toxic to cells. This can lead to fevers, night sweats, chronic fatigue, joint pain, skin sensitivity, rashes, swelling, reduced mobility, heart problems, palpitations, pain, double vision, loss of vision, eye pain, photosensitivity, etc. If the infection persists it can lead to hepatitis of the liver, spinal meningitis, peripheral neuropathy, and paralysis; and if it gets into the brain, it can cause cerebral meningitis, a very serious condition that is difficult to reverse. Chronic Fatigue Syndrome and Fibromyalgia have overlapping symptoms and may be part of the same illness process. Mycoplasma infection is often misdiagnosed as Multiple Sclerosis or Amyotrophic Lateral Sclerosis (often called Lou Gehrig's disease).[33]

Our clinical experience has revealed that many patients with cancer of the reproductive organs, liver or breast have dental granulomas (cysts), decay, or root canals in the corresponding teeth, heavy-metal toxicity and/or high dental electrical readings and pathogenic mycoplasma. These same patients have a life-long history of associated symptoms like headaches, numbness, ringing in the ear, electrical currents in the face and head, chronic sinus infections, facial pain, heart irregularities, panic and anxiety, depression, joint pain and chronic fatigue. Many health practitioners and their patients learn the hard way that therapeutic progress is difficult to achieve if there is a bacterial infection in the jaw that is suppressing the immune system. Therefore, if you have metal fillings, or had any teeth extracted, or have root canals, you should be aware that toxins from dental infections are hidden killers.

Traditional dentistry, as practiced in the United States, has been slow to acknowledge the health hazards of using mercury as a dental filling and does not always consider the relationship between the teeth and the health of the whole body. There is an alternative, however, and that is Biological Dentistry.

Biological dentistry is a holistic approach to dental health that acknowledges that dental work affects not only the teeth, gums and jaw, but also influences the entire body and health of the individual. Pioneered in Germany over 25 years ago, Biological Dentistry focuses on treatment and therapies that are non-toxic, bio-compatible and supportive of the immune system.

Using thermographic, physiologic and bioresonance methods to locate chronic areas of disease, Biological Dentistry corrects problems caused by hidden or residual infections, necrosis and chronic inflammation. Biological Dentistry also addresses the chronic health effects from the release of toxic metals from non-compatible fillings and prostheses.

When heavy metal toxicity is determined to be a contributing factor behind a serious health problem it is important that the removal of these dental fillings be done safely. A Biological Dentist is trained to assess the overall health of the patient before removal and detoxification. When mercury fillings are not removed properly additional contamination can occur due to the vapors released from the drilling. Mercury particles from the filling can also be released into the mouth and swallowed. This only makes the toxic burden worse. A Biological Dentist uses a "rubber dam" to prevent the patient from swallowing any of the amalgam particles. He or she also administers oxygen to prevent the patient from breathing mercury vapors from the drilling and to keep mercury vapors from escaping into the sinus cavities or into the brain. A good Biological Dentist will perform the removal over several appointments to avoid stress to the immune system. Intravenous vitamin C infusions during the removal procedure facilitate mercury processing and excretion by the body. For the safe and effective removal of mercury from the tissues it is advised to work with a Biological Dentist trained in the protocols as outlined by Dr. Hal Huggins, DDS. There are several internet sites, including www.NaturalHealingHouse.com, devoted to this subject.

Once the offending metals have been removed a good Biological Dentist tests the replacement filling material for bio-compatibility. Just because the dentist offers porcelain fillings doesn't mean that your body is not going to have an allergic reaction to the synthetic compounds in the porcelain or to the bonding material.

It is important to find a Biological Dentist that is trained to see granulomas and cavitations on x-rays and has experience in treating these issues in a holistic and effective manner. Your life can depend on it.

Scalar Heart Connection™

You have just explored 14 principles for optimal physical health and vitality. There may be more, but these are the primary principles that we have found to be the most important in our clinical experience. We used to think that there is an emotional component in most of our chronic illness cases. Recently, we have come to the conclusion that there is an emotional component in ALL cases of degenerative illnesses. For this reason, we always start with every client at the level of inner connection and positive mental and emotional attitude. We use two basic tools to help people change the resonant frequency of their negative perceptions or the cellular memory of traumatic events. The first is Holographic Repatterning, which you were introduced to in Principle #2. The second tool is called Scalar Heart Connection. This is based on the principles of scalar waves introduced in Principle #1 and takes advantage of the body's ability to generate its own source of scalar waves.

Our ability to create a high scalar potential through the activation of our built-in circulatory möbius coil provides us with the opportunity to move the energy 'potential' into action through our intention. It is as though the standing scalar field is waiting for our instruction. It can remain as a field of unlimited potential, or the potential can be put into action by our will to act.

Take a moment to consciously breathe into the chest and feel the tingling in your lungs and throughout the body created by this increase in energy. Now visualize this standing field of potential energy waiting for your instruction. You can direct this scalar energy, through intention, to go anywhere in your body that needs energy (healing). If you have an area of pain or disease you can focus your intention of healing on this area. You can focus your attention/intention inwardly to connect or strengthen any weaknesses you feel about yourself or anything else you are thinking about that weakens you. A 'correction' is the process of identifying the limiting or weakening thought, feeling, issue, or disease and consciously using the unlimited potential of your own scalar waves to cancel the negative frequencies they create and replace them with positive, life-enhancing frequencies through your intention to do so.

Energy healers use tuning forks, toning, color therapy, etc., to introduce corrective healing frequencies into the body/mind system of their patients. These are all aimed at stimulating or enlivening specific needed frequencies that are missing, muted or out of phase (off tune). All of these modalities affect the scalar heart center through intention.

When energetic connections are aimed at the scalar heart center, you energize and enliven the two central energy channels that flow along the midline of the body and through the heart. The first channel is called the Conception Channel, which runs along the midline in the front of the body. The second channel is the Governing Channel, which runs along the midline in the back of the body. When energetic connections are aimed at the scalar heart center, you affect these two channels, which in turn energize the other specific organ and system meridian channels as found in traditional Chinese acupuncture.

Scalar Heart Connections also stimulate any desired changes along the spinal cord, activating the nervous system, the quantum energy matrix, the brain and our consciousness. These connections can change all of our energetic systems and physical systems. They also affect mental, emotional, psychological, psychic and spiritual patterns.

We instruct all of our clients on how to make Scalar Heart Connections for themselves at home. This helps support and strengthen them against the adverse effects of negative thoughts and opens the door to the journey of self-healing. The Scalar Heart Connection can be done in six steps:

1. Start by consciously breathing in slowly and deeply, visualizing the breath coming in as golden white light through the top of your head. This will activate the pineal gland, which is situated at the center of the brain and is suspended in a chamber filled with water (cerebral fluid). The pineal acts as an oscillator receiver and transmitter. As a receiver we are able to tune into the stillness of the quantum field of unlimited potentiality. As a transmitter, we can transmit our 'intention' throughout our body through the cerebral spinal fluid, reaching every cell of our body.

2. Visualize the golden white breath being transmitted from the pineal gland into the möbius coil within the major heart scalar center. Each time you breathe in you

are now filling the lungs with oxygen, which is rich with electrons. By increasing the amount of electrons in the lungs, you are strengthening the scalar wave generation by the heart and vascular system. The lungs act like a scalar wave battery or storage center. Continue to breathe into this area slowly until you feel "full" or maybe even a bit light-headed.

3. Visualize the mobius coil configuration of the heart getting brighter and brighter with golden white light. Next, imagine yourself getting smaller and smaller until you can see yourself inside the royal chamber of your heart. See yourself seated on the throne of your heart, surrounded by the unlimited power of scalar waves.

4. From this position you can look out over your kingdom below. "See" and "feel" where there is an area in the matrix of your kingdom that is not coherent. Is there an area of pain or suffering?

5. Find the feeling behind this non-coherent pattern. You need to find the fear behind that which generates the feeling. The sense of separateness drives fear, fear of the unknown, fear of failure, fear that we are not loved. Fear is the result of not understanding that we are not separate from the very source of who we are.

6. As the Master of your kingdom you are empowered to command the scalar waves to strengthen and correct the matrix for this feeling/fear/negative belief. Do this by using your scalar waves to reset the matrix. Remember, your scalar waves not only give command

or intention to the möbius coil of the heart but this extends to the möbius coils within the mitochondria (cell energy factories) of every cell in your body. Many people find it helpful to make a motion with their hand upwards and towards the heart and say "connection" to reinforce the intention.

In Conclusion

The way we feel about ourselves and how we react to outside stimuli directly affects how we receive energy and how well our body communicates energy to every cell. The quantum, scalar field of unlimited potential is the background that connects all of us to ourselves, to each other and to the universe. This energy is the blueprint that directs and regulates all biological processes. In order for this energy to manifest as physical health we must ensure that we are providing our body with all the necessary nutrients needed by our cells—the most basic and fundamental component of our "physical" manifestation.

We can view the energy of information and regulation as being like musical notes on the conductor's score. Each note tells the musicians in the orchestra of our body what notes to play. The conductor is the regulator that tells the musicians when to play the notes, how long, how loud, and when to stop. This is like the cell membrane sorting out incoming signals from the environment and our thoughts and directing DNA to send instructions for protein synthesis. If there is any disruption on this energetic communication level the sound coming from the orchestra will not be pleasant or beneficial.

But this is only one side of the equation. The orchestra members won't be able to play beautiful harmonious music if they receive all the right notes and direction from the conductor but they don't have functioning instruments. It is just as important that we provide our cells with the nutrients they need to carry out DNA instructions and other cellular functions. If DNA is the instrument and it is damaged due to free radicals then instructions for protein synthesis will not be received or communicated. Likewise, if the inter- and intra-cellular fluid is acidic or toxic then the enzymes needed for protein synthesis or hormone communication will become deactivated. In both cases the result is cellular degeneration, leading to fatigue, chronic illnesses and premature death.

True healing comes about when we address the bio-energetic level and the physical level together. It requires a holistic and integrative approach. Physical health and vitality is the end result of integrating these two concepts and making them a part of our daily lives.

References

1) Chang, J.J.; Fisch, J.; Popp, F.A., *Biophotons*, Kluwer Academic Publishers, 1998.

2) Popp, F.A.; Nagle, W.; Li, K.H.; et al., *Biophoton Emission: New Evidence For Coherence and DNA as Source*, Cell Biophysics 6:33-51, 1984.

3) Kamenetskii, F., *Unraveling DNA*, Perseus Books, 1997.

4) Rein, G., *The Body Quantum: Non-classical Behavior of Biological Systems*, "The Resonance in Residence Science Addendum," Ilonka Harezi, 2002.

5) Lipton, B., Insight Into Cellular Consciousness, *Bridges*, 2001, Vol 12(1):5

6) Wolff, M., *Tetrode and EPR: Matter Waves and Buddhist Thought.*

7) Lipton, B., *The Biology of Belief*, 2001

8) Wordsworth, C.F., *Holographic Repatterning Modalities for Transforming Resonance Patterns*, Wordsworth Productions, 1994.

9) Wentz, M., *Invisible Miracles*, Medicis, S.C., 2002.

10) Morter, TM, *Fell's Official Know-It-All Guide—Health & Wellness*, Fell, 2000.

11) Giampapa, V.C.; Yanick, Jr., P., *Pro-Hormone Nutrition*, Longevity Institute International, Montclair, New Jersey, 1998.

12) Murray, M.; Pizzorno, J., *Textbook of Natural Medicine*, Livingstone, 1999.

13) Yanick, P., *Quantum Medicine*, Writer Services Publications, 2000.

14) Jensen, B., *The Chemistry of Man*, Bernard Jensen International, 1983.

15) Holford, P., *The Optimum Nutrition Bible*, The Crossing Press, 1999.

16) Campbell, T.C., *A Plant-Enriched Diet and Long-term Health, Particularly in Reference to China*, Paper presented at the Second International Symposium on Horticulture and Human Health, Alexandria, VA, (November 4, 1989).

17) Campbell, T.C., et al., *China: From Diseases of Poverty to Disease of Affluence. Policy Implications of the Epidemiological Transition*, Paper part of NIH Grant R01CA33638 (Bethesda, Md.: National Institutes of Health, 990).

18) Malkmus, G., "Caffeine, a Dangerous Drug", *Alive Magazine*, January 2002.

19) Weintraub, S., *Monosodium Glutamate and its Many Forms*.

20) Tirtha., *The Ayurveda Encyclopedia; Natural Secrets to Healing, Prevention and Longevity*, Ayurveda Holistic Center Press, Bayville, New York, 1998.

21) Batmanghelidj, F., *Your Body's Many Cries For Water*, Global Health Solutions, 2001

22) Baldwin, K., The Therapeutic Value of Light and Color, *Let There Be Light*, by D. Dinshah, Third Edition.

References

23) Nick, G.L., Addressing Human Exposure to Environmental Toxins with Chlorella pyrenoidosa, *Townsend Letter for Doctors & Patients*, April 2003.

24) Reiss, U., *Natural Hormone Balance for Women*, Pocket Books, 2001.

25) Weindruch, R., *Caloric Restriction and Aging*, Scientific American, January 1996, 1, 46-52. 2000.

26) Nick, G.L., *Dietary Restriction: A Fundamental Key to Supporting Detoxification and Ensuring Health and Longevity*, Townsend Letter for Doctors & Patients, November 2000.

27) Bowman, C., *Electromagnetic Fields A Danger, Scientists Say*, The Sacramento Bee, October 18, 2002.

28) Ziegler, J., "Immune System May Benefit from the Ability to Laugh", *Journal of the National Cancer Institute*, pg. 342-343.

29) Oschman, J., *Energy Medicine, the Scientific Basis*, Churchill Livingstone, 2001.

30) Meinig, G.E., *Root Canal Cover-up*, Bion Publishing, Ojai, California, 1998.

31) Kasprzak, K.S., *Nickel in Genotoxic and Carcinogenic Metals: Environmental and Occupational Exposure*, Fischbein, L. Furst; Princeton, N.J., 1987.

32) Linsteadt, S.M., "New Applications in Identifying Platelet Markers of Chronic Illnesses", *Townsend Letter for Doctors & Patients*, January 2003.

33) Nicholson, G., CFIDS Awareness Conference, June 1, 1997.

Resources

Natural Healing House

- Natural support for those with cancer or other chronic illnesses—herbal formulas, poultices, German homeopathics, heavy metal detoxification, etc.

- Quantum Healing Codes™

Telephone: (866) 300-5243
www.NaturalHealingHouse.com

Lectures / Seminars / Workshops

- The Heart of Health: The Principles of Physical Health and Vitality

- Scalar Heart Connection™

Telephone: (866) 300-5243
www.NaturalHealingHouse.com

Holographic Repatterning

Telephone: (505) 533-6060
www.holographic.org

Pharmaceutical-grade Cellular Nutrition

Telephone: (530) 477-6956
www.unitoday.net/naturalhealing

Notes: